The Royal Marsden Hospital
Manual of Standards of Care

The Royal Marsden Hospital Manual of Clinical Nursing Procedures Third Edition

560 pages, illustrated paperback
ISBN 0632 033878

Edited by A. Phylip Pritchard and Jane Mallett

This manual guides nurses in the application of the latest research findings thus ensuring that theory and practice are integrated.

The Royal Marsden Hospital Manual of Clinical Nursing Procedures has been extended and updated throughout. New procedures have been added thereby maintaining its contribution to the development of excellence in nursing and nurse education. It has also been adopted by a number of health authorities as a basis for their nursing procedures.

Key features are:
- research-based guidelines
- all procedures are accompanied by rationale
- in line with developments in education
- valuable to nurses at all stages of their careers
- versatile- can be used with many nursing models
- procedures are arranged in alphabetical order for quick reference
- clear illustrations enhance the text

Every procedure has two sections

1. Reference Material: consisting of a short review of the literature and other relevant material. A list of references and further reading is included at the end to indicate the source of the information and to assist the reader to follow up the topic if more detail is required.
2. Guidelines: this section provides a list of the equipment needed, followed by a detailed step-by-step account of the procedure and the rationale for the proposed action.

Some procedures have a third section devoted to nursing care plans, giving a list of the problems that may occur, their possible causes and suggestions for their resolution.

Contents
Abdominal paracentesis; Arterial lines; Aseptic technique; Barrier nursing; Nursing the infectious or immunosuppressed patient; Bladder lavage and irrigation; Bone marrow procedures; Bowel care; Cardiopulmonary resuscitation; Central venous catheterization; Continent urinary diversions; Cytotoxic drugs: handling and administration; Discharge planning; Drug administration; Enteral tube feeding and nutritional assessment; Entonox administration; Epidural analgesia; External compression and support in the management of chronic oedema; Eye care; Gastric lavage; Intrapleural drainage; Intravenous management; Iodine-131 treatment protocol; Last offices; Lifting; Liver biopsy; Lumbar puncture; Mouth care; Neurological observations; Observations; Oxygen therapy; Pain assessment; Peritoneal dialysis; Perioperative care; Scalp cooling; Sealed radioactive sources; Specimen collection; Stoma care; Syringe drivers; Tracheostomy care; Traction; Transfusion of blood and blood products; The unconscious patient; Urinary catheterization; Venepuncture; Violence: prevention and management; Wound management.

For further information please contact
Nursing Books Department on (01865) 206206

The Royal Marsden Hospital Manual of Standards of Care

Edited by

Joanna M. Luthert
MSc, RGN, H Dip HV
Onc Cert Quality Assurance Officer

and

Lorraine Robinson
BSc (Hons), RGN
Onc Cert Lecturer in Cancer Nursing

**Blackwell
Science**

© 1993 The Royal Marsden Hospital

Blackwell Science Ltd
Editorial Offices:
Osney Mead, Oxford OX2 0EL
25 John Street, London WC1N 2BL
23 Ainslie Place, Edinburgh EH3 6AJ
350 Main Street, Malden
    MA 02148 5018, USA
54 University Street, Carlton
    Victoria 3053, Australia

Other Editorial Offices:

Blackwell Wissenschafts-Verlag GmbH
Kurfürstendamm 57
10707 Berlin, Germany

Zehetnergasse 6
A-1140 Wien
Austria

First published 1993
Reprinted 1995, 1997

Set by Best-set Typesetters Ltd, Hong Kong
Printed and bound in Great Britain at
the University Press, Cambridge

The Blackwell Science logo is a trade mark of Blackwell Science
Ltd, registered at the United Kingdom Trade Marks Registry

DISTRIBUTORS
Marston Book Services Ltd
PO Box 269
Abingdon
Oxon OX14 4YN
(*Orders:*   Tel: 01235 465500
             Fax: 01235 465555)

USA
Blackwell Science, Inc.
Commerce Place
350 Main Street
Malden, MA 02148 5018
(*Orders:*   Tel: 800 759 6102
             617 388 8250
             Fax: 617 388 8255)

Canada
Copp Clark Professional
200 Adelaide Street, West, 3rd Floor
Toronto, Ontario M5H 1W7
(*Orders:*   Tel: 416 597 1616
             800 815 9417
             Fax: 416 597 1617)

Australia
Blackwell Science Pty Ltd
54 University Street
Carlton, Victoria 3053
(*Orders:*   Tel: 03 9347 0300
             Fax: 03 9347 5001)

A catalogue record for this title
is available from the British Library

ISBN 0-632-03386-X

Library of Congress
Cataloging-in-Publication Data

The Royal Marsden Hospital manual of standards of care / edited by
  Joanna M. Luthert and Lorraine Robinson.
    p. cm.
  Companion v. to: The Royal Marsden Hospital manual of clinical
nursing procedures.
  Includes bibliographical references and index.
  ISBN 0-632-03386-X
  1. Hospital care – Standards – Handbooks, manuals, etc.
  2. Hospital care – Quality control – Handbooks, manuals, etc.
  3. Royal Marsden Hospital (London, England) – Handbooks, manu-
als, etc. I. Luthert, Joanna M.   II. Robinson, Lorraine,   III. Royal
Marsden Hospital manual of clinical nursing procedures.
  [DNLM: 1 Royal Marsden Hospital (London, England)
  2. Hospitals – standards – England.   3. Quality Assurance, Health
Care – England. W 84 R8]
  RA972.R69   1993
  362.1'1'0218421 – dc20
DNLM/DLC
for Library of Congress   92-49009
                                                          CIP

Contents

Foreword

I am very pleased to have been asked to write the foreword to the first edition of *The Royal Marsden Hospital Manual of Standards of Care*. This Manual represents a considerable achievement in defining the excellence in practice to be achieved by members of the multidisciplinary team to offer the patient with cancer the best quality care.

The implications of this at the present time in the post-White Paper Health Service could not be more apparent. Both the providers of care and those purchasing health care to meet the needs of patients with cancer will find this Manual invaluable in determining the levels of care to be achieved to ensure that patients with cancer receive care that is both efficient and effective – meeting their often complex needs at the first attempt.

The Manual, however, not only defines quality care, but also describes how to measure the achievement of quality – so ensuring that the search for quality becomes an ongoing issue – and a very real issue for staff at all levels within a health care organisation.

Comments and suggestions from those who use the Manual will ensure that the ongoing, dynamic nature of defining quality in cancer care is perpetuated and debated and these will be included in any further editions.

Robert Tiffany, OBC
Director of Patient Services
Chief Nursing Officer

Introduction

In 1989 The Royal Marsden Hospital began an initiative to define standards of care determined by a range of health care professionals – chaplains, dietitians, nurses, occupational therapists, physiotherapists, social workers and speech and language therapists. These standards were to be used as the basis for measuring the quality of care provided to patients and their relatives – highlighting areas that required the implementation of change to ensure that care of the highest quality was offered.

Four years later the initiative continues and this Manual presents the work that has been completed to date. The initiative is an evolutionary one. The examples of standards and auditing tools in Parts Two and Three of the Manual are not definitive, they reflect the current position at the time of publication.

The Royal Marsden Hospital is a Postgraduate Special Health Authority specializing in the care of patients and their relatives with cancer. The standards and auditing tools will reflect this interest, but contain material that has a wider remit and are underpinned with philosophies of care that every health care organization should strive to emulate.

The information provided in Part One is designed to assist the reader to take the standards and auditing tools and adapt them to their own health care environment with imagination and interpretation. The standards and auditing tools are designed to be amended: firstly, to reflect the problems and needs of patients or clients and their relatives wherever they are receiving care; secondly, the needs of the professional groups providing care; and finally, the needs of the health care organizations to produce information relating to the quality of services offered to their patient population.

Part Two of the Manual presents examples of the standards, and Part Three the auditing tools produced by the individual members of the multidisciplinary team. They are arranged alphabetically by discipline and then alphabetically again according to the subject of the standard or audit.

The Manual is designed to be a companion to *The Royal Marsden Hospital Manual of Clinical Nursing Procedures* and is cross referenced with this publication wherever appropriate.

Acknowledgments

Our attempts to acknowledge all the contributions to this text will necessarily fall short. We are indebted to all the health care professionals whose views, opinions and clinical expertise were the mainstay of the project and without whose enthusiasm and commitment we would not have been able to start, let alone complete this manual.

We extend our special thanks to Mr Robert Tiffany (Director of Patient Services/Chief Nursing Officer) for his continued advice and support, and to Miss Lindsey Pegus (Head of Medical Art Department) for her assistance. We also thank Mrs Lynda Warner for her thoughtful and critical comments and development of the auditing tools.

Finally our thanks to Lisa Field and her colleagues at Blackwell Science Ltd for their encouragement and patience.

J.M.L.
L.R.

PART ONE

QUALITY ASSURANCE – DEFINING AND MEASURING QUALITY

1

Quality Assurance – Process, Management and Practice

Introduction

This chapter defines and describes the concept and the process of quality assurance. The economic, political and professional pressures and influences to define and then measure the quality of care and services provided to patients are identified. The chapter also identifies the need to develop a quality management structure that incorporates the key principles of a 'bottom-fed top-led' approach supported by an effective communication system and responsive leadership. Putting this into practice is the next stage, for without this basis quality assurance initiatives will not only lose credibility but the risk is that nothing will happen to alter the quality of care and services provided to patients.

The practicalities of the quality assurance programme established within a health service organization are described – the strategy followed to implement the 'bottom-fed top-led' approach within the organization – and the scene set for one of the major quality initiatives being undertaken within the organization – the Nursing and Rehabilitative Therapists Audit initiative. The initiative is put into perspective as one part of a detailed and comprehensive quality assurance programme that provided staff at all levels of the organization with a matrix of quality information upon which decisions could be made relating to the possibility and desirability of change.

Definitions of quality and assurance

Defining quality is difficult – it is a concept – it is a notion, an idea, an abstraction. The *Concise Oxford Dictionary* definition suggests that it is a 'degree of excellence' (*Concise Oxford Dictionary*, 1982). It is a subjective concept, as Pirsig comments in *Zen and the Art of Motorcycle Maintenance* (1974): 'quality is what you like'.

It is also an elusive concept. Brooks (1989) suggests

that: 'quality is a moving target – a process of continuous improvement', and continues to suggest, pessimistically, that quality is 'a prize to be coveted, if only ever to be imperfectly achieved'.

The pressures are present however, to turn this subjective, elusive and unattainable concept into something objective, graspable and both possible and desirable to achieve. To that end the concept has to be made practical, translated into a process – an activity – that starts by defining 'quality' and 'excellence' clearly, concisely and comprehensively so it can then be measured to provide evidence of achievement or otherwise. This process forms the basis of all quality assurance initiatives.

The word 'assurance' is defined as 'a formal guarantee ... certainty' (*Concise Oxford Dictionary*, 1982). Quality assurance initiatives should, therefore be so designed that they provide a formal guarantee that a defined degree of excellence is being achieved.

In practice the process of quality assurance follows the model shown in Fig. 1.1. The process begins with the definition of the level, or degree, of excellence to be achieved. It continues with the measurement of whether or not this level of excellence has been achieved. At this stage the process divides. If the level of excellence has been achieved there are two options. Firstly to check that the defined level of excellence was set at the appropriate level – can the target be moved? If so, the level of excellence must be redefined. Or secondly, if the level is to stay the same, the measurement phase can continue.

If the desired level of excellence has not been achieved the next stage in the process is to identify the deficits, the problems or difficulties that are making that level of excellence unattainable. Once these are identified, consideration must be given to whether change to achieve the target is either possible or desirable. If it is, change must be implemented and

3

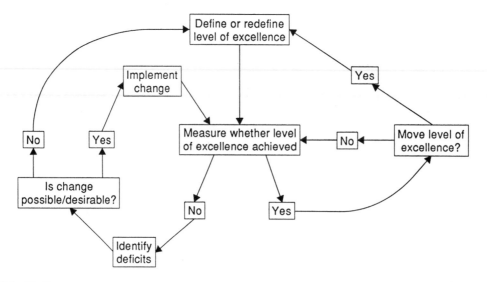

Figure 1.1 Quality assurance process.

the process continues with reassessment. If, however, for whatever reason change is not possible or desirable the stated level of excellence must be redefined.

It is through following this process of events that the concept of quality and the process of quality assurance becomes an everyday activity. Quality assurance has become an activity that affects all the members of the multidisciplinary team involved in patient care and the consumers of health care. Quality assurance initiatives take on a number of guises: there are the professionally focussed initiatives such as medical, nursing and rehabilitative therapists' audit; or organizationally focussed initiatives such as in-patient satisfaction surveys, where environmental and non-professional issues are assessed. The publication of 'The Patients Charter' (1991) has drawn the attention of the consumer to the 'degree of excellence' – the quality – they should expect and experience within health care organizations.

The reasons for the drive to monitor and assess the quality of care and services provided within health care organizations are complex. Understanding the reasons and being aware of the stimuli and the underlying influences allow health care professionals to use quality assurance initiatives to their and their patients' advantage; to capitalize both professionally and politically to ensure that care of the highest quality is both attained and maintained.

Quality assurance – the economic and political context

The economic pressures to evaluate the quality of care and services provided within the National Health Service are not necessarily new, but health care has changed beyond recognition since the beginning of the century and even over the last decade or so. This has prompted the need for assessment and evaluation.

There have been technological advances and associated alterations in the demand for health care and health services – advances in scanning techniques to facilitate more accurate diagnosis, surgical advances with the increasing use of laser surgery and microscopic techniques both of which have resulted in faster throughput of patients, reduced in-patient time, increases in day surgery and faster discharges (International Society for Quality Assurance in Health Care, ISQA, 1989). There are also epidemiological and social changes which affect health care provision and delivery, an increase in the elderly population with pathological consequences such as increasing reporting of senile dementias (Adams & Duchen, 1992) and the advent of previously undiagnosed disease processes such as HIV, the human immuno-deficiency virus (Vlahov, 1989).

These changes have stimulated the need to assess health care provision, rationalizing services and resources and offering services that are cost-efficient and effective. There will always be a finite limit to the resources available to finance and support health care services and, inevitably, the achievement of quality care will be determined by such constraints. It is achieving a balance that is acceptable both for the provider and the receiver of health care services that is pivotal to the debate.

The work of health care professionals has changed considerably and new roles and functions have been developed in line with the new technologies and demands (ISQA, 1989). Health care organizations are large structures employing personnel in a number of specialist capacities. There is a risk that each specialist group works in isolation from the others – care may become fragmented and the differing personnel may become marginalized and isolated within the health care organization. The contribution and specialist function of members of the team may be questioned – and more cost-effective replacements may be identified. Duplication of roles and activities are clearly not cost-effective, nor is the use of highly trained and expensive health care professionals to perform tasks for which they are over qualified. This can become an issue for some professional groups as alternatives for their expertise and skills are identified – the introduction of health care assistants for example, to fulfil some of the roles and functions of professionals such as nurses and physiotherapists.

Patient behaviour and expectations have changed over the past decades. The image of the compliant, non-questioning patient is changing as patients are beginning to challenge all aspects of their care – from the skills, expertise and attitudes of the health care professionals to the environment and non-technical aspects of care such as cleanliness, privacy and punctuality (Annual Report of the Health Service Commissioner, 1990–91; Which? Way to Health, 1991).

The definition of patients as 'consumers' of health care or as 'customers' may feel uncomfortable to some health care professionals, but it is the reality in the 'new' post White Paper Health Service of the 1990s (DoH, 1990). 'The Patients' Charter' (DoH, 1991) encourages all citizens to be aware of their National Health Service rights and to question when these rights are not realized. Legislation ensures that wherever a patient or relative formally questions the care received, an investigation is initiated and will continue until the patient or relative is satisfied with the information or assistance provided (Hospital Complaints Procedure Act 1985). The Data Protection Act 1984 and the Access to Health Records Act 1990 have formalized access to health records – thereby facilitating questioning and examination of the care provided.

The culture of health care organizations is changing, but perhaps the most catalytic change has been the implementation of the National Health Service and Community Care Act 1990.

The National Health Service and Community Care Act 1990 'split' the health service into purchasers and providers. The basis of communication between the two groups are contracts; contracts that specify what is to be provided, at what cost, to whom and with what guarantees of quality. Quality is identified as a fundamental part of the contracting system and purchasers are encouraged to request evidence of:

'the provision of systems to assure quality such as medical, nursing and other audit and surveys of patient opinion'

(DoH, 1990)

The National Health Service Management Executive have been careful to emphasize that purchasers do not overlook quality in their quest for value for money:

'the contractual process should be directed to improving the quality of services provided and not to efficiency and cost-effectiveness alone'

(DoH, 1990)

The central objectives and ideologies supporting the recent reforms of the Health Service are the achievement of quality and a genuine desire to put the patient first:

'behind the policies of the White Paper lies the important question of quality and the extent to which our systems, processes and facilities put the patient at the centre. Success in these areas is not easily achieved. It requires positive and continuous effort, led from the top, which puts patients – our customers – at the centre, and is built on wholehearted support by every staff group and at every level within the organisation' (Nichol, 1989a).

The stimuli and the influences to assess care and services are not only economic and political; they are also a part of the values held by health care professionals. Such professionals share the ideologies expressed in the above quotation – where the patient is the centre of care delivery, where quality of care is seen as being of paramount importance and where these beliefs are shared and supported by all members of that professional group.

Response of the professional groups

The professional groups within the Health Service have responded and reacted to the economic and political pressures. Systems to evaluate aspects of care, particularly in nursing, have been advanced and used for some considerable time with varying degrees of success (Pearson, 1987). The Royal College of Nursing took a professional lead in the definition of quality for nurses with the 'Standards of Care Project' (Royal College of Nursing, 1989) and the establishment of the 'Dynamic Standard Setting System' (Royal College of Nursing, 1990). The rehabilitative therapists have also identified professionally-led strategies for the measurement of quality and have determined professional standards of care for their patient groups (College of Occupational Therapists, 1989; Chartered Society of Physiotherapists, 1990 and College of Speech and Language Therapists, 1991).

Systems for auditing nursing and rehabilitative therapists care have been advanced and supported financially by the National Health Service Management Executive (1991). It is not inconceivable that audit of the quality – and inherent in this process the assessment of cost-effectiveness and efficiency – of the work performed by nurses and rehabilitative therapists will become statutory in the same way as medical audit (Health and Health Care Research Unit, 1990).

Auditing – checking and examining aspects of professional practice, following the stages of the quality assurance process – is an activity with which the professional groups within health care organizations are well acquainted. Evaluation of care has always been integral to professional practice. The emphasis now is on formalized and comprehensive evaluation – providing evidence to demonstrate that quality care is, or is not, being both attained and maintained.

The quote from Duncan Nichol (1989a) raises other issues for the professional groups within the Health Service: issues that are crucial to the application and support of systems to measure quality of care. The issue of leadership is fundamental as is the issue of 'whole hearted support . . . at every level of the organization'. There are certain key principles that must be considered if the auditing of care following all the stages of the quality assurance process is to be accomplished. These are principles that apply to both to the management of the process and to the management of the information that is produced as a result.

The management of quality

There are three factors that are essential to ensure the success of any quality assurance initiative – from definition of quality, to measurement, to the implementation of change. These factors relate directly to the concepts of leadership and staff participation suggested by Nichol (1989a) and form the basis of a quality management structure:

- Ownership
- Communication
- Leadership.

Ownership

Firstly, it is essential that the health care professionals who are at the hub of patient care are the people determining 'levels of excellence', defining quality. This not only promotes professional credibility and endorsement of the level of excellence that is to be achieved, but also fosters a sense of 'ownership'.

Many quality assessment tools are criticised for adopting a 'top-down' approach – where levels of quality are defined either externally to the organization, or by managers within the organization who are removed from the day-to-day reality of the clinical situation, and where the tool is implemented by managers or external assessors rather than being defined and implemented by or in consultation with staff (Harvey, 1990). The consequence of initiatives where this is the approach may be that the health care professionals are alienated and dissociated not only from the results of the assessment but also from their organization. They may be being asked to conform to a level of excellence that they had no part in determining, and which they did not agree that they could achieve.

If change for the better is the preferred outcome of such an exercise the fostering of a sense of ownership is fundamental and is a critical part of the management of change within organizations (Porter *et al.*, 1987). Strategies for change resulting from quality assurance initiatives should also be determined by those at the centre of patient care and those strategies then discussed and negotiated with the relevant managers of the service.

Communication

The second factor is the establishment of a responsive two-way communication system within the health care organization between those at the centre of patient care and those at the most senior levels of management who hold ultimate responsibility for the quality of care and services offered to patients. The communication system must disseminate information about the quality assurance initiatives that are being implemented, the results from them and the options for change where this is indicated. This ensures not only that the level of excellence defined by those at the hub of patient care is shared and endorsed throughout the organization, but that the results of quality assurance initiatives are also shared and acknowledged.

In practice, this involves the identification and maintenance of a well developed and sensitively managed exchange of information at all stages of the quality assurance process that flows both upwards and downwards, as well as laterally, to ensure that everyone involved at every stage of the process shares and participates in the initiative.

Leadership

Management support at all levels of the organization may be required to facilitate change – particularly where there are resource or policy implications for the achievement of excellence. This forms the basis for the third principle, that of leadership. The end point in the communication chain needs to be either an individual or an identified group who has the power invested within them to motivate, support and, if necessary, insist on strategies for change if these are indicated as a result of quality assurance initiatives.

There is a balance to be struck between managers and those at the centre of patient care. Managers within the organization need to be aware of the importance of consultation and negotiation with staff, and of being seen to participate actively in the quality assurance process themselves in order to facilitate the process of change (Porter *et al.*, 1987). Just as ownership by the health care professionals at the hub of patient care is identified as fundamental, so is influential and powerful leadership from the top. In practice the quality assurance process must be 'bottom-fed' and 'top-led' with an effective and well developed communication system in operation.

Nichol (1989a) identifies two points that further support the need to have a defined model of the management of quality based on this 'bottom-fed top-led' approach. These are, firstly, the stimulation of 'positive and continuous effort', and secondly 'whole-hearted support'. Neither of these concepts are realizable without some form of quality management structure and without effort and support quality

will only ever be 'imperfectly achieved' (Brooks, 1989).

Quality management in practice

In practice the management of quality within our health care organization evolved over time, responding to the variety of pressures and influences discussed previously. The organization had appointed a Quality Assurance Officer who was responsible for quality initiatives within nursing and rehabilitation before the implementation of the National Health Service and Community Care Act 1990. Nursing care had been assessed on a regular basis for some time to collect evidence related to both the quality of services provided and the efficiency of such services.

The political pressures to assess the quality and efficiency of all care and service provision became more apparent as the National Health Service prepared itself for the National Health Service and Community Care Act 1990. In 1989 a directive was sent by the National Health Service Management Executive to all Regional, District and Postgraduate Special Health Authority General Managers that determined priorities for quality assessment activities (Nichol, 1989b). The directive encouraged health care organizations to appoint a key worker for quality initiatives and to focus on establishing priorities for quality monitoring.

The Quality Assurance Officer became the key worker throughout the organization with the responsibility to co-ordinate and implement hospital-wide quality assurance initiatives. A Quality Assurance Group of senior managers was established to support the Quality Assurance Officer. The management of the organization was not based on a clinical directorate system, but on a system of directorates designated according to function (as shown in Fig. 1.2).

The group consisted of the Director of Patient Services – responsible for nursing and rehabilitative therapists; the Director of Clinical Services – responsible for medical care and technical services such as pharmacy and radiography; the Director of Operational Services – responsible for hotel, catering and portering services, and responsible for responding to patients' letters of complaint and praise; the Director of Personnel – with a responsibility for staff and staffing issues; the director responsible for contracting and planning; and the Quality Assurance Officer.

The group met regularly and had both a strategic

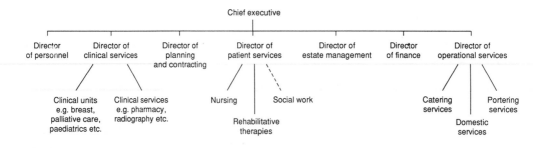

Figure 1.2   Management structure (simplified diagram).

and an operational brief. The strategic brief was to determine priorities for quality assurance initiatives, support such initiatives and then act on the results to facilitate change. The operational brief was to participate in quality assurance activities, to be seen by staff to be actively involved and to take an interest in quality issues. The group was accountable to the Chief Executive and to the Hospital's Management Executive to whom the results of major initiatives were presented.

As the role and function of the Quality Assurance Group developed so a Quality Assurance Team evolved. Members of the team were responsible for the various quality assurance initiatives being developed and implemented. The team consisted of two permanent members – the Quality Assurance Officer and an Assistant Quality Assurance Officer – but included other members as and when initiatives and funding were identified. National Health Service Management Executive funding was obtained to finance a position within the Quality Assurance Team for the Nursing and Rehabilitative Therapists Audit initiative. The team was accountable through the Quality Assurance Officer to the Chairman of the Quality Assurance Group.

Once a quality assurance initiative was identified for development the Quality Assurance Team would work closely with the relevant staff at the centre of care or service delivery to determine the best way to implement the quality assurance process. This group of staff would then take on the responsibility for determining strategies for action if, after the measuring phase of the process, the need for change was identified. The members of these 'Quality Improvement Groups' were personnel with a managerial responsibility to ensure that change could and would be considered and then implemented wherever possible. For example, the Quality Improvement Groups of a clinical unit would be representative of all

the health care professionals providing care to that patient population – speech and language therapists, dietitians, nurses – and increasingly, the medical staff, who welcomed the opportunity to discuss quality related issues as a full multidisciplinary team.

The Nursing and Rehabilitative Therapists Audit initiative followed this format at the measurement and implementation of change stages in the quality assurance process. The definition stage required another level of interaction – a level that would provide the initiative with objectivity and credibility. The initial phase of this initiative involved members of each professional group within the multidisciplinary team determining levels of excellence for clinical care. Levels of clinical excellence were determined, therefore, by practising experts within each professional group who had day-to-day experience of the issues they were confronting.

Where the definition of quality required obtaining the views of a number of staff within the professional groups, 'Consensus Groups' were established. The Consensus Groups were facilitated by a member of the Quality Assurance Team and represented all the differing grades or expertise of staff having day-to-day experience of patient care. The manager of the service would then represent that professional group at the clinical unit multidisciplinary Quality Improvement Group, and was responsible for ensuring that quality related information was communicated to all members of his or her professional team. The Consensus Groups did not have a managerial remit; their function was to ensure that the definitions of quality reflected the majority view in terms of both acceptability and attainability.

This quality management structure is represented in Fig. 1.3. The factors identified as being essential to the achievement of quality are deeply enmeshed within the structure. The 'ownership' of quality initiatives was established at Quality Improvement Group

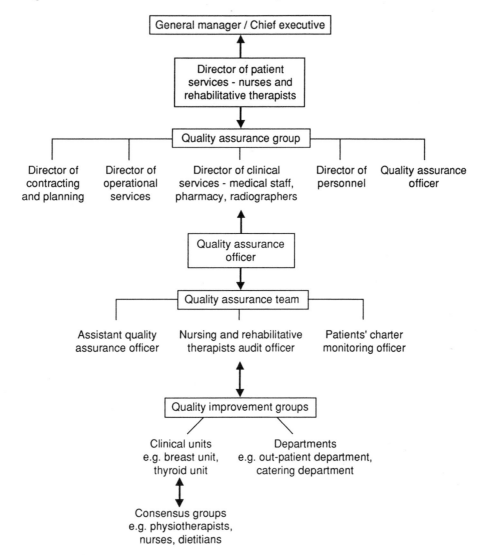

Figure 1.3 Quality management and communication structure.

level, or at Consensus Group level where this was appropriate. It was at these two levels where quality of care and services were defined, measurement systems identified and agreed upon and strategies for action were then drawn up and implemented. This was the 'bottom-fed' part of the structure. The 'top-led' element was also in place with the formation of the Quality Assurance Group – the members of which had the authority and influence to support the range of quality assurance initiatives and to facilitate change. The communication system was facilitated through

the Quality Assurance Team and through the Quality Assurance Officer whose role it was to co-ordinate and implement quality assurance initiatives throughout the organization and who was a member of the Quality Assurance Group.

Providing a matrix of quality information
The quality assurance initiatives included in the organization's operational plan covered a wide variety of the care and services provided not only to patients but also to staff. The Nursing and Rehabilitative

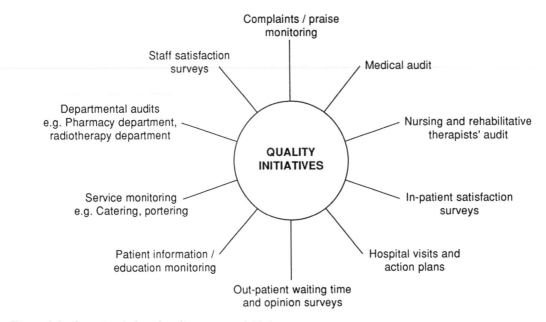

Figure 1.4 Operational plan of quality assurance initiatives.

Therapists Audit initiative was one part of the quality assurance programme which was developed to provide staff at all levels of the organization with a matrix of quality information. The information provided used a variety of sources, a variety of methods and a variety of perspectives to provide staff with a multidimensional view of the quality of care or service they were providing. This information could then be used to decide whether change was desirable or possible and to determine strategies and priorities for such change. Many of the initiatives examined the provision of non-clinical care and services and focussed on the environment in which care was provided. This needed to be balanced with the ability to assess the quality of clinical services – in such a way that the needs and requirements of the patients, the health care professionals and the health care organization were met.

The pressures were there – economic, political and professional. The process by which it could be done was identified and the structure was in place to facilitate, support and maintain it. The framework was in place – now was the opportunity to run with it.

References

Adams, J. H. & Duchen L. W. (Eds) (1992) *Greenfield's Neuropathology*, 5th edn, Chapter 20. Edward Arnold, London.

Annual Report of the Health Service Commissioner: 1990–1991 (1991) HMSO, London.

Brooks, T. (1989) *Best of Health: Winning Entries for the Hospital of the Year 1989*. Sunday Times Andersen Consulting Health Care Practice, London.

Chartered Society of Physiotherapists (1990) *Standards of Physiotherapy Practice*. Chartered Society of Physiotherapists, London.

College of Occupational Therapists (1989) *Standards of Practice for Occupational Therapists 1–6*. College of Occupational Therapists, London.

College of Speech and Language Therapists (1991) *Communicating Quality: Handbook of Standards of Care*. College of Speech and Language Therapists, London.

Concise Oxford Dictionary of Current English (1982). 7th edn, Clarendon Press, Oxford.

Department of Health (1989) *Working for Patients*. HMSO, London.

Department of Health (1990) *Working for Patients: Operational Principles*. HMSO, London.

Department of Health (1991) *The Patient's Charter*. HMSO, London.

Harvey, G. (1990) *Which Way to Quality. A study of the implementation of four quality assurance tools. A summary report. Royal College of Nursing Standards of Care Project*. Institute of Nursing, Oxford.

Health and Health Care Research Unit (1990) Clinical Audit in Professions Allied to Medicine and Related Therapy Professions: *Report to the Department of Health on a Pilot Study*. The Queen's University of Belfast, Belfast.

International Society for Quality Assurance in Health Care (1989) Editorial. *Journal of Quality Assurance in Health Care*, **1(1)**, 1.

Kitson, A. (1989) *Standards of Care: A Framework for Quality*. Royal College of Nursing, London.

National Health Service Management Executive (1991) *Framework of Audit for Nursing Services*. Department of Health, London.

Nichol, D. (1989a) *National Health Service Management Executive Management Bulletin, Issue 28*. Department of Health, London.

Nichol, D. (1989b) Circular EL(89)/MB/117. National Health Service Management Executive. Department of Health, London.

Pearson, A. (Ed) (1987) *Nursing Quality Measurement: Quality Assurance Methods for Peer Review*. John Wiley, Chichester.

Pirsig, R. (1974) *Zen and the Art of Motorcycle Maintenance*. Corgi, London.

Porter, L. W., Lawler, E. E. & Hackman, J. C. (1987) *Behaviour in Organisations*. McGraw-Hill, Singapore.

Royal College of Nursing (1990) *Dynamic Standard Setting System*. Royal College of Nursing, London.

Vlahov, D. (1989) AIDS: overview, immunology, virology and informational needs. In *Seminars in Oncology Nursing*, **5(4)**, 227–35.

Which? Way to Health (1991) *Complaining to the NHS*. Consumers' Association, London.

Acts of Parliament

Access to Health Records Act 1990.

Data Protection Act 1984.

Hospital Complaints Procedure Act 1985.

National Health Service and Community Care Act 1990.

2

Defining Quality – Standard Writing

Introduction

Chapter 1 described the quality assurance process – the stages of defining quality, measuring it and then implementing change where this was identified as being necessary. The structure for managing quality was also described and the role and function of Quality Improvement Groups and Consensus Groups discussed. This chapter focusses on the first stage of the quality assurance process – the definition of quality – and describes the way in which quality care was defined by the members of the multidisciplinary team – chaplains, dietitians, nurses, occupational therapists, physiotherapists, social workers and speech and language therapists. Examples of the resulting standards of care are presented in Part Two.

The theoretical basis

Two sources were used as the theoretical basis for writing the standards of care. The two sources were the works of Donabedian (1966) and Wilson (1987).

Donabedian wrestled with the problem of defining the quality of medical care in the United States of America in the 1960s. He described the measurement of effective medical care in terms of 'structures, processes and outcomes'. 'Structures' included the adequacy of health care facilities, the qualifications of practitioners and the financial aspects of medical care. 'Processes' were the aspects of care that demonstrated that 'medicine is properly practised', and 'outcomes' the concrete and precise measurements of the effectiveness of medical care – survival rates, restoration of function and so on.

Wilson's (1987) contribution to the debate on how to define quality was to take these definitions and operationalize them into something tangible and practical. Wilson redefined Donabedian's model as 'inputs; methods or procedures; and outcomes'. Wilson elaborated further to describe inputs as

'people, equipment and environment' – the resources required to attain a defined level of care. Methods or procedures became the everyday practice that was required – the professional or technical skills or expertise. Outcomes were targets of care or services as measured by 'productivity, quality and client satisfaction'.

These two theoretical sources were fused together to form the basis for writing the standards of care presented in this Manual. The synthesis of the two sources is represented in Fig. 2.1. Donabedian's 'structures' became Wilson's 'inputs' and for our purposes became 'resources' – what the health professional required access to in order to achieve the defined level of excellence. Resources included the three categories defined by Wilson – people, equipment and environment. 'Processes' became 'methods or procedures' and then finally became 'professional practice' – what the health professional did in order to achieve the defined level of quality care. Outcomes remained as outcomes throughout the models, combining both Donabedian and Wilson in terms of efficiency, effectiveness and satisfaction.

The stated outcomes of care were the consequences of efficient and effective use of resources and the following of professional practice. This was assessed in terms of evidence of satisfaction of both the patient and the health care professional with the results of the health care strategies and evidence from the documentation system.

Wilson offered definitions of 'standard' and 'criteria' – two words which were often used interchangeably and with confusing consequences with Donabedian's 'structure, process and outcome'. Wilson stated that a 'standard' was 'a definition of attainment' and 'criteria' were 'the smallest of a hierarchy of definitions of performance'. For our purposes a 'standard' was taken as being the

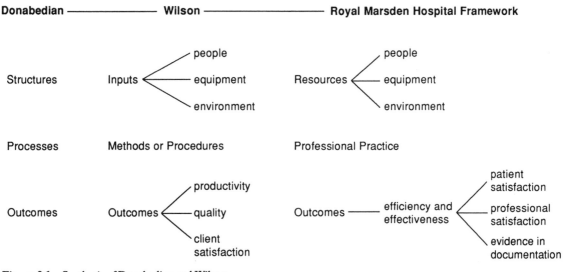

Figure 2.1 Synthesis of Donabedian and Wilson.

entire document that was produced when quality was defined and then delineated further into the three sections outlined. 'Criteria' were taken as the individual items defined within these three sections.

Producing a framework for defining standards of care became straightforward once these two sources were combined and an understanding was reached on the meanings applied to key words.

The framework
A framework was established that was used by all the health care professionals involved in producing standards of care. The framework followed the pattern outlined in the proceeding sections (it may be helpful to refer to an example of a standard from Part Two while the component parts are described).

Standard statement
The standards began with a clear and concise definition of the level of excellence to be achieved for a patient with a specific problem or need – by the specific member of the multidisciplinary team. This was a statement of intent – the 'Standard Statement' (Kitson, 1989) and incorporated key aspects of practice that were to be achieved in the care of a patient with this defined problem or need.

Rationale
The definition of the level of care to be achieved was supported with a researched and referenced rationale describing clearly and concisely the extent and nature of the need or problem and justifying the input of that specific professional group.

Resources
The resources required to achieve the defined level of care were categorized under the three sub-headings suggested by Wilson (1987):

- People
- Equipment
- Environment.

People
The 'people' criteria of the resource section included the baseline knowledge and skills that the health care professional required. The knowledge and skill criteria would be expected to be included as a part of professional education and training programmes either at first level training or as part of post-basic or specialist education. The health care professional would also have access to continuing education either as part of in-service training arranged by the manager of the service or through access to externally run educational programmes to both maintain and further develop their knowledge and skill base.

The 'people' section also included a list of the other members of the multidisciplinary team who were identified as essential to act as a resource for both the health care professional and the patient if this level of care was to be achieved.

Aspects of the role and function of the manager of the professional group were also summarized within the 'people' section. The manager was identified as a resource to members of their own professional group as well as to other members of the multidisciplinary team as an identified clinical expert. The responsibilities of the manager to provide educational and professional support for staff were also clearly identified. These requirements were identified as crucial to the ability of the health care professionals to achieve excellence in practice.

Equipment

The 'equipment' criteria of the resource section included both specialist and non-specialist items that were seen as essential to the provision and achievement of quality care. Items such as syringe drivers for the management of chronic pain, availability of specialist speaking tubes for insertion into tracheostomies to facilitate speech production following a laryngectomy and so on. In the standard relating to the management of a patient with anorexia this section included the availability of teaspoons for patients to eat yoghurts and ice cream, for example, as there was a shortage of this particular item at ward level and they were necessary to fulfil aspects of professional practice.

The section included the provision and availability of written information for patients – admission information booklets, exercise information sheets, or booklets on aspects of treatment or side-effects of therapy – and access to written information for staff, such as policy and procedure manuals (Pritchard & Mallett, 1992).

Environment

The 'environment' section included a description of the environment that, wherever possible, should be made available for the patient and which would reflect his or her individual needs and requirements. This might include information about the provision of an area designated and equipped for physiotherapy treatments, or the provision of an area of privacy in which aspects of care or treatment could be discussed.

The environmental needs of the professional group were also included in this section – the requirement to have access to an area for completing clerical work, access to clean, well lit areas for the preparation of drugs and so on.

Professional practice

The professional practice section of the documents described in detail the assessment, planning, implementation and evaluation of care that were the integral parts of every health care professional's activity to manage the identified need or problem. The section was not intended to be so detailed as to be prescriptive – personalized care remained the central objective with the flexibility to plan care to meet individual needs and requirements. The section did need, however, to include sufficient detail to ensure that critical elements of assessment, planning, implementation and evaluation of care were clearly described.

Specific aspects of professional practice were also stressed – such as information giving, and providing explanations of proposed care, teaching and educating the patient in practical skills where appropriate to facilitate independence, and providing emotional support and comfort.

Within this section the nurses were identified as the co-ordinators of care and communicators of information to other members of the team where their initial assessment or subsequent evaluation would lead them to decide to make a referral. The standards written by the other members of the multidisciplinary team included referral guidelines to ensure that referrals were made appropriately both in terms of the management of the need or problem but also in terms of the optimum time to facilitate the best outcome for the patient. Patient-centred care was stressed throughout the professional practice sections encouraging involvement of the patient in all aspects of care wherever appropriate and practical.

Documentation of all aspects of professional practice was regarded as an essential part of the process – not only to ensure continuity of care and to demonstrate professional accountability, but also for auditing purposes. The development and implementation of multidisciplinary care plans facilitated this process. These care plans were designed to permit a detailed first level assessment of the patient on his or her first contact with the health care organization. The assessment was performed by the nurse practitioner responsible for the patient's care. Using the information gained from it, the nurse identified the problems or needs specific to that patient and the appropriate members of the multidisciplinary team to implement the necessary health care strategies. The problem or need was identified within the documentation system and each member of the multidisciplinary team recorded the actions taken to implement the agreed health care strategy in the one document.

Outcomes

This section of the standard document delineated the expected results of the health care strategy, and indicated in broad terms what evidence should be sought to indicate that this level of care had been attained.

This would include evidence of efficiency and effectiveness assessed in terms of patient and professional satisfaction and documentary evidence. Evidence that the standard had been achieved would be provided from all three sources through information relating to resource availability and use and the following of key aspects of professional practice.

The outcome section of the standards, therefore, defined the expected outcomes of the management of a patient's problem or need from three perspectives:

- Patient opinion – that they were satisfied with the care they received.
- Professional opinion – that they were satisfied with the care they provided.
- Documentary audit – that there was evidence of access to and timely use of resources and that key aspects of professional practice were followed.

Each component part of the standard related to another. The outcome section of the standards was the common link back to each of the preceding sections, and reflected the complex inter-relationships between defining the level of quality to be achieved, defining the necessary resources and professional practice and then defining the outcomes to be expected as a result of achieving that level of care.

Identification of standards

The subjects for the standards were identified either by searching the documentation system for the most frequently occurring patient problems or needs, or through discussion with each professional group to determine commonly presented patient problems.

The rehabilitative therapists wrote 'general' standards of care that described an overall level of quality to be attained for patients receiving rehabilitative care from a specific discipline, and delineated the baseline knowledge and skills each professional group required together with referral guidelines and so on. More specific standards of care related to clinical areas such as palliative care or rehabilitation following breast surgery evolved from these general standards, but this general, non-specific information was not repeated.

The nursing standards reflected a diverse spectrum of clinical care. Where a clinical unit had an identified area of nursing expertise the standards produced by

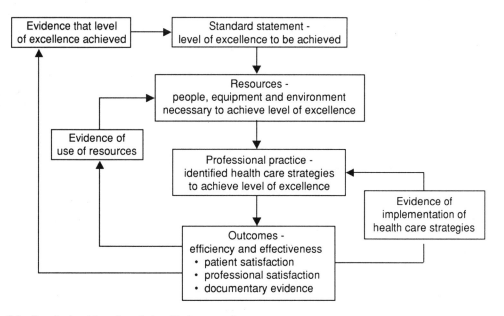

Figure 2.2 Standard writing: the relationship between the component parts.

that unit were used, wherever appropriate, throughout the health care organization. This prevented duplication and encouraged consistency of clinical care from one unit to another.

The standards were written independently by members of the multidisciplinary team. This was a deliberate decision taken at the outset of the initiative to allow for acknowledgement of the differentiation of input between health care professionals. The end point of care was often the same for all the members of the team but the route by which a patient was facilitated to achieve the outcome by the various health professionals was often very different. For example, the outcome of the management of pain for all health care professionals was to alleviate or contain it – but the health care strategies adopted by physiotherapists, occupational therapists, nurses and chaplains to achieve this were all different.

The complex interrelationships between all the members of the multidisciplinary team were acknowledged in each of the standards where other members of the team were identified as a resource to the patient or to the health professional. Wilson (1987) noted that in 'human service work' it is difficult to attribute accurately the efforts of an individual or a professional group, but there was a need for each member of the multidisciplinary team to be able to define his or her own specialist input to the overall wellbeing of the patient.

Ownership, communication and leadership

Ownership of the standards was achieved through Consensus Groups which were formed to write the standards of care once the subjects had been agreed upon. These Consensus Groups were groups of health care professionals representing all the differing grades or expertise within that profession. They were facilitated by a member of the Quality Assurance Team – the Nursing and Rehabilitative Therapists Audit Officer. All the members of the Consensus Groups had day-to-day experience of the range and complexity of patients' problems or needs to be addressed and defined.

Once the standards were written a process of review and communication was initiated. The standards were reviewed by managers to ensure that they reflected a level of quality that was achievable within the resources available. Aspects of the standards relating to education and training were also checked to be sure that they reflected a realistic and achievable educa-

tional level for the health care professionals, and that the criteria were covered by formal and informal educational programmes. Wherever possible the standards were also reviewed by experts in the appropriate field – experts within the same or another professional group. This process assessed the 'state of the art' accuracy of professional practice and also monitored potential professional duplication or overlap of roles and functions.

Once these preliminary reviews had taken place the standards were presented to the Director of Patient Services (the senior manager within the directorate) and to the Patient Services Committee (the policy and planning committee of the directorate). The standards were presented to this committee by a member of the Quality Assurance Team and a representative of the appropriate Consensus Group. Comments from the committee would be negotiated and then incorporated into the standards to ensure that they reflected achievable targets of excellence that would then be supported throughout all management levels.

Once agreed the standards were returned to the clinical units and departments and put into a 'Quality Manual'. Every unit and department built up a manual unique to its clinical area containing a selection of relevant standards from all the members of the multidisciplinary team.

This system of review and ratification at the definition stage of quality care ensured that the three factors identified as key to the success of quality management – ownership, communication and leadership – were well established before progressing to the measurement phase of the quality assurance process and the implementation of strategies for change. This process is a part of the Quality Management Structure described in Chapter One, and is an elaboration of this system within one directorate to facilitate the 'bottom-fed top-led' approach.

The implications of defining standards

There were a number of implications of defining standards beyond measuring the quality of nursing or rehabilitative therapists' care. Defining levels of excellence and then delineating the resources and professional practice required and the expected outcomes of care had other significant ramifications. The three major implications of defining quality care were as follows:

- Managerial
- Educational
- Professional.

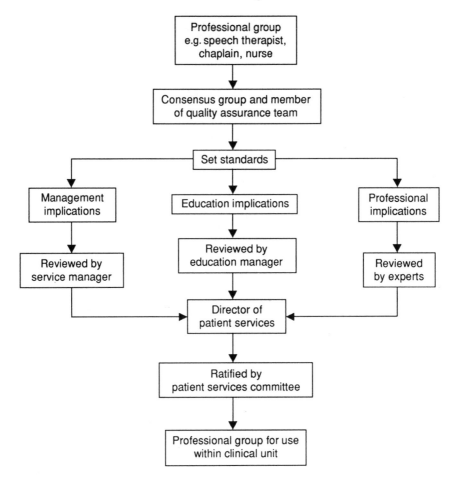

Figure 2.3 Review and ratification process.

Managerial implications

The delineation of resources had implications for managers within the health care organization. Listing the equipment that was required to achieve a certain level of care, and describing the optimum environment within which care was provided to patients, had resource and budgetary implications. Care had to be taken to ensure that the standards were achievable and realistic – reflecting the constraints within the organization – yet sensitive enough to highlight deficiencies in resource provision where this was prohibiting the achievement of the agreed level of care.

Some aspects of change would also require management support – not only financial – in the allocation, or reallocation, of resources to increase manpower, to purchase additional equipment, or to finance or organize further educational training for staff for example. Management support would also be necessary to change aspects of professional practice which involved changes in policy or negotiations with the managers of other services within the organization.

Educational implications

The standards had educational implications at a number of differing levels. Firstly, having a manual of standards available at ward or department level was an educational tool for staff new to the area, or staff who needed to identify the most appropriate member of the multidisciplinary team to refer a patient to, or the key areas to assess the patient for with a specific problem or need, for example. Standards produced incorporating this amount of detail were a guide to all aspects of assessment, planning, implementation and evaluation of care.

The detail that was offered in these documents fulfilled a second educational implication – that of providing information for the development of educational curricula and competency levels. By delineating the knowledge and skills required of the practising professional to achieve a given level of care it was possible to extract elements required of both formal and informal educational programmes. The knowledge and skills criteria plus the professional practice section contained valuable information about what was to be expected of members of the professional group – from those responsible for the day-to-day delivery of care to those in management positions.

As these standards were defined by practising members of each professional group – by those at the hub of patient care – those members of the organization were influencing educational curricula and clinical competencies rather than having these determined for them. This was an exciting development.

Professional implications

The professional implications related to the power that these documents had in terms of identifying what it was that individual members of the multidisciplinary team did in their everyday practice. Our experience was that producing documents of this kind increased a sense of professional confidence and self-worth for all team members.

The importance of articulating the professional responsibility and the professional expertise required in the planning and delivery of care of the highest quality had never been more evident. In an environment of accountability and rationalization of service provision to ensure that care was competitive and represented value for money, the roles and functions of every member of the multidisciplinary team were under the spotlight. Documents such as these and the evidence produced from auditing care were important in defending the input and impact of each and every member of the team wherever it demonstrated that excellence was the end result.

Producing evidence was the next stage – developing the auditing tools to accompany each standard that would examine the expected outcomes of care in more detail using the three sources of evidence (the patient, the professional and the documentation system).

References

Donabedian, A. (1966) Evaluating the quality of medical care. *Milbank Memorial Fund Quarterly* **XLIV**, No 3, Part 2, 166–203.

Kitson, A. (1989) *Standards of Care: A Framework for Quality*. Royal College of Nursing, London.

Pritchard, A. P. & Mallett, J. (1992) *The Royal Marsden Hospital Manual of Clinical Nursing Procedures*, 3rd edn. Blackwell Scientific Publications, Oxford.

Wilson, C. (1987) *Hospital Wide Quality Assurance: Models for Implementation and Development*. W.B. Saunders, Ontario.

3

Measuring Quality – Auditing Standards of Care

Introduction

In Chapter Two the framework for writing standards was described and the relationship between the component parts of the standards discussed. The relationship was stressed between the expected outcomes of care and all the other sections of the document – the standard statement that defines the level of care to be achieved, and the resources and professional practice necessary to attain this.

The outcomes of care reflected the expected consequences of efficient and effective care from three perspectives – the perspective of the patient, the perspective of the health care professional and the documentation of care. Stating the outcomes of care only fulfilled the first part of the quality assurance process; the next stage was to measure whether these outcomes were being achieved in practice. The standards defined quality but did not measure it, auditing tools needed to be developed from the documents to enable this process.

Designing the audit tools

The auditing tool for each standard consisted of three questionnaires. The three parts of the auditing tool were aligned to the three perspectives identified for the outcome criteria:

- Audit of patient opinion
- Audit of professional opinion
- Audit of documentation.

The auditing tools for each standard were developed wherever possible with the same consensus group and the managers of the units/departments that originally defined that standard. The inclusion of the managers was seen as important for two reasons. Firstly, they had expert status in that area of care or service delivery and could focus on key issues in the assessment of the delivery of care. Secondly, they were account-able for the care or service provided within their unit/department and so the results of the auditing initiative had to provide them with the information that they, as managers of that service, would find useful.

The source of questions for the auditing tools derived from the standard statement and the expected outcomes, and all three questionnaires focussed on the availability and use of resources and the following of professional practice. The questions were designed to assess the efficiency and effectiveness of care in terms of patient and health care professional satisfaction and documentary evidence. The finer detail was provided by the nature and content of the patient problem or need that the standard was addressing. Examples of the auditing tools are included in Part Three.

Audit of patient opinion

The questions in this section of the audit tool related to resource availability and use, but focussed predominantly on professional practice. The outline areas for questioning were as follows:

- Was the problem/need resolved or contained by the professional group?
- Was the level of support appropriate?
- Was the level of information appropriate
- Were the family able to be involved in care if they wished to?
- Were adequate preparations made for discharge – advice, support, practical assistance?
- Overall, was the patient satisfied with the care provided?
- What were the most and the least helpful aspects of care?

The questions were a mixture of closed yes/no style questions with space to add additional comment and open-ended questions about the more general aspects of the care or services provided. The questionnaire was designed to be completed by the patient, or by a relative if this was appropriate.

Audit of professional opinion

The questions in this audit tool focussed on both resource availability and access and to professional practice. There were five outline areas for investigation:

- Was the problem/need resolved or contained?
- Were the necessary people, equipment and environment available?
- Was professional practice followed?
- Did the health care professional perceive that the patient was satisfied?
- Was the health care professional satisfied?

The questions were closed yes/no questions, but additional comment was invited. This questionnaire was designed to be completed by the health care professional who had day-to-day responsibility for the care of the patient whose care was the subject of the audit.

Audit of documentation

The audit of documentation questionnaire contained questions relating to access and use of resources and professional practice and covered these seven outline topics:

- Was the patient assessed for key issues relating to the problem or need?
- Did the health care strategy address these issues?
- Was the patient offered help and support to manage the problem/need?
- Was the patient provided with necessary information?
- Were appropriate and timely referrals made to members of the multidisciplinary team?
- Was the health care strategy evaluated and was the strategy altered accordingly if this was indicated?
- Was the problem/need resolved or contained?

All these questions were closed yes/no style questions. This section of the audit tool was designed to be completed by the health care professional with day-to-day responsibility for the patient together with the manager or a senior member of that professional group.

The questionnaires were to be as short and succinct as possible, focussing on key issues, and so rarely exceeded ten questions unless this was genuinely felt to be necessary. This decision was based on the very practical reason of time: time for the patient, time for the health care professionals involved in the process and time involved in the turn-around of information gained from the initiative. The more detailed the audit the longer it would take to collect, collate and analyse the data from the questionnaires and return it to the manager for interpretation and action.

The design of the audit tools was an ongoing process, testing and retesting, trying out different formats. This work is still continuing. The practical application of the audit tools is also an area that continues to be refined. The initiative is an evolutionary one.

Practical application of the auditing tools

Each unit or department had access to a Quality Manual which consisted of a selection of the standards and associated auditing tools representing the patient problems or needs presented on that unit/department. A topic for audit was chosen from this selection by the manager of the unit or department in conjunction with the Quality Assurance Team. There were a number of practical issues that had to be discussed and agreed with the manager and the staff of the unit/department before care could be audited.

Preparation of staff

Preparation of the staff on the unit or in the department was crucial. The concept of ownership at the measurement stage in the quality assurance processs was as important as at the definition stage. A member of the Quality Assurance Team would meet the staff whose care was to be the subject of audit together with the manager to discuss the practicalities of the audit and to answer any questions that the staff might have. Reducing staff anxiety was a primary concern, monitoring performance was stressful, careful preparation and time for discussion appeared to reduce this. Encouraging staff to see the exercise as positive and constructive rather than negative and critical was the key. The role of the manager was also critical, their attitude to the initiative could make or mar the whole process. Encouraging involvement and wholehearted participation by the whole team overcame most difficulties.

Sample size

Determining the sample size to audit was an obvious practical consideration. The maximum number of patients chosen as an auditing sample was 20, but it could be as large or as small as was felt to be manageable so long as the size of the sample reflected some degree of accuracy of representation of the patient population being examined. The sample could also be determined by some other criteria other than numbers of respondents. It could be determined by time, for example, auditing every patient with the chosen problem or need over a fixed period of, say, two weeks or three months. One unit chose to audit every patient with a given clinical problem over the course of one day.

Twenty patients were chosen as the maximum number to audit for practical reasons. Twenty patients would generate a maximum of 60 completed questionnaires to collect, collate and then analyse. The managers also found that staff enthusiasm began to wane after six weeks of data collection and this had to be taken into consideration.

Encouraging both staff and patient participation was critical in maximizing the highest response rate with small sample populations. The evidence from other patient opinion initiatives undertaken in the health care organization suggested that the response rate was likely to be good, and as with these other initiatives considerable efforts were made to inform and explain the audit of care to the patients. At the top of each questionnaire was a brief explanation to the patient explaining why this initiative was taking place and inviting and encouraging patient participation. Patients were also reassured that any information would be treated confidentially; a sealable envelope was provided to place the completed questionnaire into and no details were requested on the questionnaire that would facilitate their identification. This protection of anonymity was also extended to the staff invited to offer their opinions about the care they were able to provide as a part of the audit.

Patients for the audit were identified from the documentation system. The titles of the standards reflected the language used in the documentation system to identify patient problems or needs.

Timing of the audit
The timing of the audit was dependent on the nature of the specific problem or need. For short term, acute problems the optimum time was at the resolution of the identified problem or need. For longer term, chronic problems the audit could be done at any stage of the implementation of the appropriate health care strategy and this provided useful information relating to the management and containment of the problem

over time. The timing of the audit was an issue that was discussed and agreed with the manager and the staff of the unit/department.

For some professional groups, it was appropriate to perform the audit at the end of a course of out-patient treatment – physiotherapy following breast surgery, for example. For others the most appropriate time was at the end of an in-patient admission when a major problem or need had been addressed – the dietetic care of a patient following major head and neck surgery, for example. It might also be performed at the end of one of a series of in-patient admissions where the patient was having cyclical treatments or investigations – the nursing care of a patient experiencing an alteration in body image such as hair loss or change as a result of chemotherapy, for example.

The unit that chose to monitor the quality of care for one specific clinical problem over the course of one day collected information at all stages of the management and containment of that problem. It was important in this instance to collect additional information for interpreting purposes – information relating to the stage of the management of the problem for each patient being audited.

Duration of the audit
Although the topics for audit were chosen from commonly presented problems, it was also important to audit problems that occurred infrequently. The audits could be divided into 'slow track' (infrequently occurring problems) and 'fast track' (frequently occurring problems). Fast track audits of a maximum of 20 patients could be completed relatively quickly – depending on the frequency of presentation and identification of the specific problem or need. Slow track audits could take considerably longer. One unit audited a specific area of patient care that only presented once a week. It was feasible to run a slow track and a fast track audit at the same time within a unit or department.

A standard was audited every three to six months in each unit and department. The frequency of auditing was left flexible to accommodate the time lags in collection of information, the collation and presentation of the data produced, and then the time required for implementing any changes and reassessing aspects of care delivery if this was necessary.

Completion of the questionnaires
In the examples cited the patient questionnaire was given to patients while they were in hospital – either as

in-patients or as out-patients. The out-patients were provided with a pre-paid envelope in which to return their completed questionnaire, while the in-patients were asked to complete the questionnaire at whatever stage of their admission was appropriate for the collection of the auditing information. The in-patients were provided with a sealable envelope in which to return their completed questionnaire.

Auditing care in this way raised important issues: issues of patient compliance balanced against the cost of audit, the introduction of bias and the accuracy of information collected. There were the cost considerations of sending a questionnaire to a patient's home rather than giving it to them while in the organisation and the costs of providing pre-paid envelopes in which to return the completed questionnaire. There was also the risk that the response rate may be more variable with a postal style survey where the response rate can be less than 50% (Hoinville & Jowell, 1987). This had to be balanced against the evidence that patients may only feel able to comment negatively (if this is what they want to do) from the security of their own home rather than from the exposed position as an in or out-patient, and that it may also be that a few days after discharge they have a clearer perception of what were good and bad experiences for them (Hoinville & Jowell, 1987).

The wording and tone of the explanation to encourage patients to participate in the audit was critical, together with the promise that all information was confidential and would be treated as such. The explanation that was used was as follows:

> 'The *physiotherapy department* at The Royal Marsden Hospital are constantly trying to improve the service they provide to patients. It is of enormous help to have the views of patients to help us do this and we would like to collect some information from you about your experience of the care the *physiotherapists* provided.
>
> We would be very grateful if you would be willing to complete this questionnaire and return it in the envelope provided. The information you provide is confidential and will be treated accordingly.'

This appeared to encourage both positive and negative comment for analysis.

The identity of the person who gave the patient the questionnaire had to be considered. There was the risk of introducing bias to the response if the questionnaire was given to the patient by the health care professional responsible for their care, or by

any other member of that professional group. Where possible informed 'third parties' were identified to give the questionnaire to the patient – the ward clerk or a member of the Quality Assurance Team, for example. Patients were never placed under pressure to complete the questionnaire if they chose not to. As a further measure to protect anonymity, the completed questionnaire was returned in an envelope addressed to the Quality Assurance Team.

Requesting patient opinion and inviting comment in response to open-ended questions facilitated obtaining patient-led definitions of quality care which could then be fed in at the beginning of the quality assurance process. Up until this stage the definitions of quality were professionally-led, but once patient feedback was obtained through the audit of care the information provided could be included in redefining the standards if that was indicated (see Fig. 3.1).

The professional opinion questionnaire was completed by the member of the professional group who had overall day-to-day responsibility for the care of the patient. The confidentiality of the professional's response was maintained as carefully as that of the patient opinion questionnaire. The professional was also supplied with a sealable envelope and the completed questionnaire was returned to the Quality Assurance Team.

Time was an important element in this part of the auditing process – and this was an important part of the pre-audit briefing. The staff needed advance warning that they would need to put aside 10–20 minutes to complete this questionnaire for each of their patients being audited. The staff also required reassurance that their responses would be treated with confidence to minimize any sense of threat or anxiety.

Confidentiality was a key issue. The questionnaires were coded to preclude the need for names of the respondents to be used and for correlation purposes, but it was felt that a record should be kept of the names of patients who completed the audit questionnaires. This information was placed against the code number of the questionnaires as they were completed. The code was only able to be broken by a member of the Quality Assurance Team and the decision to do that rested with the Quality Assurance Officer. This was done if information received as a result of the initiative indicated that patient care or wellbeing was being compromised in some way. Permission of the patient was obtained by the Quality Assurance Officer to investigate an issue in more detail, for example, if information was received that required further action.

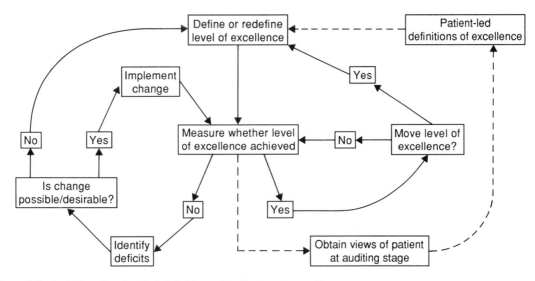

Figure 3.1 Inclusion of patient-led definitions of quality into the quality assurance process.

The multidisciplinary care plan also incorporated a section for auditing information. The date and nature of the audit was included to protect patients from frequent requests for their opinion about the care they received.

The manager of a small unit or department would need to manage the information from an audit such as this with extreme sensitivity if they were able to identify the staff responsible for the care of the patient being audited. One manager reassured her staff that audit was not personal appraisal; the information gained from this exercise was not going to be used as formal performance review. The information was to be used to determine appropriate changes in the department and not to criticize individuals.

Auditing care from these two perspectives – patient opinion and health care professional opinion – permitted and authorized these two groups within the health care organization to comment on the care they both received and provided. This appeared to facilitate a sense of empowerment for both these groups, and encouraged them to feel a valued and useful part of the health care organization.

The audit of documentation questionnaire was completed by a senior member of staff for the professional group in conjunction with the member of the team who had primary or overall day-to-day responsibility for the practical care of the patient. This part of the audit could act as a form of managerial appraisal

or performance review as well as an indicator of the quality of care provided to the patient if that was felt to be appropriate. It could serve as an informal educational exercise to review all aspects of care delivery on a one-to-one basis. This section of the audit would also take time – about 20 minutes would be necessary for searching the documentation for the appropriate information, completing the audit questionnaire and discussing any issues arising from the exercise.

There were problems for small or single-handed departments with this form of audit. One department requested assistance from a similar department from another hospital as the manager considered that as there were only three other members of her team other than herself this exercise was difficult to perform objectively. Colleagues were often willing to assist, the Quality Assurance Team were also willing to help if that was felt to be appropriate. Peer review, or internal audit of units/departments was encouraged to reduce the sense of threat to the staff involved and to maximize the concept of ownership.

Retrospective audit of health care documentation is problematic (Pearson, 1987). Health care professionals may write excellent notes but not deliver the health care strategy outlined. Alternatively, they may deliver excellent care but fail to document it. The poor standard of health care documentation is noted in the Health Service Commissioner's Report 1990–91 (DoH, 1991). It was felt that this system of docu-

AUDIT INFORMATION	DATE AUDIT COMMENCED

AUDIT INFORMATION

STANDARD OF CARE

UNIT/DEPARTMENT

DATE OF STAFF MEETING

SAMPLE POPULATION

Inclusion criteria

Exclusion criteria

Total sample

No. of questionnaires returned

DATE AUDIT COMMENCED

ESTIMATED DURATION OF AUDIT

QUESTIONNAIRES

Coding list completed   Yes [ ] No [ ]

Patient Opinion

When given to patient

Given by

Professional Opinion

Completed by

Documentation Audit

Completed by

DATE AUDIT COMPLETED

DATE REPORT COMPLETED

DATE OF FEEDBACK

ACTION PLAN AGREED

DATE OF FOLLOW UP

Figure 3.2   Example of auditing guidelines.

mentary review might serve to improve the standard of documentation, and that the staff appraisal element and managerial review might facilitate greater congruence between documented and delivered care. Once completed these were also returned to the Quality Assurance Team.

Wherever possible, all three questionnaires were completed within 48 hours while the documentation of care was available and the information relating to patient care was still fresh in the mind of the health care professional.

No greater weighting was placed on any one of the three sources of information for the auditing initiative. It was felt that the potential problems and disadvantages of collecting data from each source could be counterbalanced by this three perspective approach. In recent auditing exercises, however, members of the Quality Assurance Team have been present on the units or departments during the audit and this has provided the initiative with another perspective – that of non-participant observation. This is to be explored further as an additional method. It will need to be performed with caution, but may prove to be a valuable adjunct to the auditing methods.

Auditing guidelines were identified for each standard to provide the unit/department with the practical information they required to initiate and complete the audit. (see Fig. 3.2). The auditing initiative was seen as providing a 'snapshot' of an element of care provided to patients with a given problem or need over

STOMA CARE AUDIT

Standard Statement:

Patients who have a stoma, either permanent or temporary, will be offered support, information and practical help to enable both themselves (and their families) to care safely and independently for their stoma whilst in the hospital setting and on their return home. Nursing care will be directed towards providing a comprehensive rehabilitation programme to enable the patient to intergrate wherever possible the management of the stoma into their everyday lives.

PATIENT OPINION RESULTS

Sample size: 19   Dates of Audit: 3.92-5.92

Did you receive a booklet on stomas?

  [17] Yes
  [2] No

If yes, did you find it helpful?

  [15] Yes
  [2] No

If no, what would have made it more useful?

*   more pictures or photographs please.
*   my wife cannot read English very well - do you have translations of the book into other languages?

Did you feel that you had enough privacy when caring for your stoma?

  [11] Yes
  [8] No

If no, how could we have improved this for you?

*   The nurse and I had to talk in a cupboard - there was nowhere else to go - I'm sure that isn't right.
*   Everyone is wonderful - but I'd have liked to talk in private about all of this - the bags and everything.
*   I'd like you to have a nice room set aside for all the bits and pieces so we could have a real talk and look at things.
*   I'd take myself off to the bathroom to do my bag - but the bin to put it in was outside - so I had to carry it. Then I worried about people wanting to use the bathroom.
*   I was sorting myself out when my lunch was brought to me - I had drawn the curtains - but they just walked straight in.

Figure 3.3   Example of results of audit: (a) patient opinion.

STOMA CARE AUDIT

Standard Statement:

Patients who have a stoma, either permenant or temporary, will be offered support, information and practical help to enable both themselves (and their families) to care safely and independently for their stoma whilst in the hospital setting and on their return home. Nursing care will be directed towards providing a comprehensive rehabilitation programme to enable the patient to integrate wherever possible the management of the stoma into their everyday lives.

NURSE OPINION RESULTS

Sample size: 19   Dates of Audit: 3.92-5.92

Do you consider that you had access to all the members of the multidisciplinary team that you required to achieve this standard?

    [16] Yes
    [3] No

If no, who was not available and what impact did it have on the care that you were aiming to provide?

*   *I required information from the Stoma Care Nurse Specialist - but it was the weekend - we managed until Monday but it would have been better if someone else with their skills had been available.*
*   *The medical staff didn't decide on the site for patient's stoma until the evening before surgery - this made assessment and support difficult to achieve.*
*   *The dietitian was due to see the patient but was unwell herself - the patient was discharged without seeing her.*

Do you consider that you had access to the environment necessary to achieve this standard?

    [14] Yes
    [5] No

If no, what was unavailable or unsuitable and why?

*   *No area for privacy.*
*   *Had to talk about stoma and management behind bed curtains - I'm sure the patient felt inhibited.*
*   *We ended up talking about the stoma in the store cupboard, there was nowhere else to go.*
*   *The store cupboard is too small for all the necessary products.*
*   *The bedside lighting was inadequate, especially at night.*

Figure 3.3   Example of results of audit: (b) nurse opinion.

STOMA CARE AUDIT

Standard Statement:

Patients who have a stoma, either permenant or temporary, will be offered support, information and practical help to enable both themselves (and their families) to care safely and independently for their stoma whilst in the hospital setting and on their return home. Nursing care will be directed towards providing a comprehensive rehabilitation programme to enable the patient to intergrate wherever possible the management of the stoma into their everyday lives.

DOCUMENTATION RESULTS

Sample size: 19   Dates of Audit: 3.92-5.92

Is there evidence that the following was assessed?

			Pre-operatively	Post-operatively
a)	Patient's knowledge of what a stoma is?		[17] Yes [2] No	
b)	Patient's feelings related to the stoma?		[15] Yes [4] No	[19] Yes [0] No
c)	Patient's wishes for their family to be involved in care?		[11] Yes [8] No	[15] Yes [4] No
d)	Patient's work, leisure and social activities?	i) work	[18] Yes [1] No	[18] Yes [1] No
		ii) leisure	[15] Yes [4] No	[16] Yes [3] No
		iii) social	[15] Yes [4] No	[17] Yes [2] No
e)	Physical limitations which may affect the patients ability to care for their stoma?		[11] Yes [8] No	[18] Yes [1] No
f)	Patient/family's needs for information?	i) patient	[15] Yes [4] No	[15] Yes [4] No
		ii) family	[11] Yes [8] No	[15] Yes [4] No
g)	Condition of the stoma?			[19] Yes [0] No

Were the areas of need identified in the assessment addressed in the care plan?

[17]   Yes
[2]   No

Is there evidence that the patient was given an information booklet?

[16]   Yes
[3]   No

Figure 3.3   Example of results of audit: (c) documentation.

a fixed period of time, that could then be returned to the relevant professional group for feedback.

Collating and feeding back the results of the audit

The questionnaires provided both quantitative and qualitative data relating to the quality of care provided to the patient. The closed construction of the majority of the audit questions made collating the quantitative data straightforward. The 'yes' or 'no' responses were simply added up and expressed as totals on a blank questionnaire. The qualitative comments were typed into the appropriate section for each question on the appropriate questionnaire (see Fig. 3.3).

The collation of data was performed by the Quality Assurance Team. The team would produce a brief report for the manager and staff of the unit/department including the quantitative and qualitative data and outlining areas of immediate concern for the group to consider. The group had the opportunity to comment and add any necessary interpretation to the data – any variables that may have influenced the care given at that time – and then determine a strategy for action where this was indicated. The manager of the unit/ department discussed the strategy for action with his or her immediate manager to ensure the necessary support for the implementation of change where this was indicated, and to ensure that it was both desirable and possible within the health care organization.

The group were given a fixed period of time to respond with their initial comments and strategy for action. Their strategy included the time-frame they felt was necessary to implement any changes that were required. The team would decide with the professional group whether there was a need to re-audit parts of the standard again, and if this was the case the re-assessment would take place after the agreed time-frame. The team would also decide with the group if the definition of quality – the level of care to be achieved – needed to be redefined in line with the findings of the audit and with the possibility and desirability of change. The findings of the auditing initiative were also shared with the multidisciplinary Quality Improvement Groups for the clinical units (the management groups that represented all the members of the multidisciplinary team, including medical staff) to determine unit responses and strategies for change as a result of the findings of the audit initiative.

Further support for the implementation of change was forthcoming from the service and educational managers, who reviewed and ratified the standards, and where indicated from the Quality Assurance Group if the changes required had hospital-wide implications.

References

Department of Health (1991) *Health Service Commissioner's Report 1990–1991*. HMSO, London.

Hoinville G., Jowell R. and Associates (1987) *Survey Research Practice*. Gower, Aldershot.

Pearson, A. (Ed) (1987) *Nursing Quality Measurement: Quality Assurance Methods for Peer Review*. John Wiley, Chichester.

4

The Way Forward

Introduction

Chapters One to Three have set the scene for a major quality assurance initiative – a system to assess the quality of care provided to patients and their relatives by a range of health care professionals. The remaining sections of the manual consist of examples of the standards and auditing tools developed as the basis of this system. They are not definitive, but reflect the status of the initiative at one point in time. They are designed to be amended and adapted to suit the multiplicity of needs and requirements of a variety of patients, clients and relatives; of health care professionals and health care organizations.

Key issues have been addressed: the management of quality, promoting a sense of ownership and leadership sustained by a responsive two-way communication system, the implications of writing and measuring standards beyond simply measuring whether quality care was achieved or not, and the practical aspects of the application of auditing tools.

The initiative is not static; it continues to evolve and be refined. New ideas are triggered by the completion of one part of the initiative. A manager has an idea for adapting the system to suit a specific unit or department and that starts off another train of thought. The process is exciting and challenging at all levels of the organization. The quest for quality stimulates and focusses debate – it is inevitably an ongoing process.

There are a number of issues to be considered within the health care organization as the initiative proceeds. It is inevitable, too, that there will be issues for consideration by health care professionals seeking to implement an initiative such as this.

Issues for the future – midway through the initiative

The issues for the future correspond to the three areas described as being key: the management of quality, the implications of writing and measuring standards and the practical aspects of the application of audit tools.

Management issues

The first management issue to be considered is that of communicating with staff throughout the organization. Such communication should raise the profile of quality initiatives and ensure that staff at all levels of the organization understand the contribution they can make (and are already making) to achieve quality care and services. Members of the health care team do not work in isolation from each other, neither do they work in isolation from other departments and services within the organization. There is a complicated pattern of provider-customer relationships within every health care environment, each depending on the others for the provision of quality care and services, as well as providing quality care and services to the patient. Methods by which this aim can be achieved are:

- Firstly, educational programmes for staff within the organization to discuss the basic concepts of quality assurance and the background behind the need for initiatives of this kind
- Secondly, a system of communication such as a 'quality newsletter' that is read by staff at all levels within the organization, can be pinned onto noticeboards, circulated to staff, and which requests feedback and comments
- Thirdly, the inclusion of expected participation in quality assurance activities into all job descriptions.

This final method can be underpinned by an individual performance review system with quality issues identified as key performance indicators from the top of the organization to the hub of care and service delivery, from strategic to operational level. Feeding

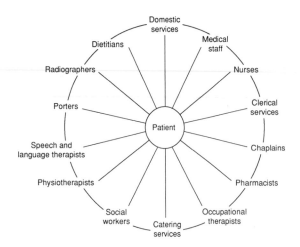

Figure 4.1 Model of provider – customer relationships within a health care organization.

back and sharing information relating to quality initiatives with patients and their relatives is another part of the educational and communication process.

The management of change following an audit of care is a major issue. Change takes time, effort and resources. The 'leaders' of the quality management structure need to support and sustain the change process; the initial audit will be seen as wasted effort if changes are identified but not seen to be acted upon, and there is no point in reauditing if some degree of change has not taken place. Honesty is crucial and constructive – if change cannot be achieved for whatever reason this must be clearly stated and agreed upon at all levels of the organization. Imaginative thinking may be necessary to achieve alternative strategies for change other than the most obvious.

The time-frame for change must also be clearly stated and staff informed if this is delayed for whatever reason. Some changes – relocating a department, for example, which includes rebuilding and refurbishing, can take a considerable time. Monitoring the change process is critical – offering assistance and support where this is indicated to sustain effort – or being more proactive and questioning and challenging why agreed changes have not occurred.

Middle-managers require support in the implementation of quality initiatives from audit through to the desired conclusion of the change process. They are caught in the centre of the process. Their units or departments may have generated information demon-

strating the strengths and weaknesses of the care or service they are responsible for providing, and then they are also held responsible for the implementation of strategies for change. If middle-managers are not supported further along the structure, they are left exposed and vulnerable with the implementation of change. The accountability for change to improve the quality of care or service provision – if that is what has been agreed – must be shared throughout the organization. Communication is the key to this, together with a responsive leadership component in the quality management structure.

Implications of audit

One of the issues that has become more apparent as the initiative has continued is that of empowerment. By being proactive in requesting both positive and negative comment, the health care organization has become more open. Requesting the opinion of both patients and staff has opened the organization externally and internally – and the organization has had to develop strategies to respond to this level of feedback.

The two key areas of development are management strategies and educational strategies. The essential components of a supportive and sustaining management strategy have been discussed in the previous section, but managers also need to learn how to respond to both the quantitative and the qualitative data, and to learn that the production and presentation of information of this kind is constructive and not destructive. Just as change in resource allocation or change in professional practice is often time-consuming, so are the changes in culture and attitude that are required to manage quality information. These issues are reflected in a report from the Audit Commission (1992):

'... organisations have to be receptive to and appreciative of criticism. This requires a cultural shift for much of the National Health Service away from a defensive style and towards greater openness about performance. Supportive management must foster an approach which accepts the occurrence of errors but which is determined to reduce them'.

The development of educational programmes to meet the needs of both patients and staff – to improve the quality and support the change of care or services provided – are an exciting advancement. Educational programmes may be necessary at all levels. These might include programmes to discuss the whys and wherefores of quality assessment (as discussed in the previous section) and then a variety of educational programmes to respond to any identified deficits in care or service provision, from professional or technical skills to customer care programmes.

Practical issues for audit in the future

There are a number of practical issues to be considered for the future. One is how to attempt to assess the reliability and validity of the audit tools used to measure the quality of nursing and rehabilitative therapists care. The initiative, as yet, has no pretensions to a scientific nature, but nevertheless changes are proposed as a result of audit of this kind. Reliability can be defined as:

'the degree of consistency with which it (the measuring tool) measures the attribute it is supposed to be measuring' (Polit & Hungler, 1987).

In practice this means that the auditing questionnaires facilitate the collection of consistent and dependable information relating to aspects of care delivery over time and from one unit or department to another, given that the same or similar circumstances prevailed. As Polit and Hungler (1987) suggest however:

'the reliability of an instrument is not a property of the instrument, but rather of the instrument when administered to a certain sample under certain conditions'.

It may be difficult to replicate the same or similar environment and circumstances to assess this accurately. There may be too many variables to contain and allow for – the situation and condition of the patient, the competence of the health care professional, the environment in which care was provided, for example. Unit-to-unit or department-to-department testing to check for reliability may also be problematic in terms of replicating the same or similar circumstances and may generate competition which is inaccurate if the audit tools are not strictly reliable.

Validity is defined as:

'the degree to which an instrument measures what it is supposed to be measuring ... are we really measuring the attribute we think we are measuring?' (Polit & Hungler, 1987).

Polit and Hungler suggest that this is often difficult to establish – particularly in psychologically oriented measures – and the measurement of satisfaction may, therefore be difficult to assess in these terms.

There are other difficulties. Asking patients to express whether their pain was reduced, or whether they felt able to manage their stoma on discharge produces subjective measures, and as discussed previously, it may also be difficult to ascribe the apparent 'success' of a particular health care strategy to one professional group. The difficulties in assessing the quality of the documentation of care have also been addressed, as this too is problematic in terms of both reliability and validity.

The addition of observation as an adjunct to the methods used to assess the quality of care is another issue to be considered and this may either help or hinder the reliability-validity debate. The presence of a non-participant observer in the unit or department may add another perspective – and the evidence from this source may contribute towards identifying whether the audit tools are collecting reliable and dependable information. Observation, however, has disadvantages related to the reliability of information that it produces as a scientific method. The difficulties with observation include the attitudes and prejudices of the observer, his or her personal interest in the situation being observed and the anticipation and hasty judgement of events that may lead the observer to describe the situation inaccurately (Polit & Hungler, 1987).

The auditing tools were designed to produce a 'snapshot' of care delivery for a given professional group, in a given unit or department, to a defined group of patients. The audit tools have been the subject of ongoing testing and retesting to assess whether the questions appear to provide an accurate response. To date, the information produced by the audit appears to be relevant and acceptable to the professional groups concerned – and has highlighted areas of change that the staff feel are warranted. It may be that this will form a part of the evidence that can be collected to assess the reliability of these auditing tools.

Another practical issue to be considered is the way in which the auditing system can be adapted to suit the needs of the health care environment, and to provide the staff with the information they require. It would be possible, for example, to audit one patient in a holistic manner by using the audit of documentation questionnaires to assess a range of problems or needs. It would also be possible to audit the care provided to one patient from all the relevant members of the multi-disciplinary team – using the professional opinion and documentation questionnaires. The permutations that the system lends itself to are open to the imagination of the health care professionals wishing to use it.

Issues for the future – at the start of the initiative

The major issues at the start of an initiative such as this are the same as those to consider mid-way through: the management issues, the implications of the initiative and the consideration of the practical application of the system.

Management issues

The first management issue is to identify the quality management structure that already exists within the health care organization and identify how to link up with it. Identifying personnel with a quality remit may be the starting point – a Quality Assurance Manager or Co-ordinator, or the manager responsible for contracts or service monitoring.

It may be useful to know what quality components are identified within contracts – how detailed the quality specifications are that relate to the provision of nursing and rehabilitative therapists' care. The business plan is another source of information about quality monitoring and how this is being implemented. The business plan may also identify other quality initiatives that are being implemented within the health care organization which may assist with linking into the matrix of quality information being generated.

Implications of audit

The primary implications of introducing an audit system to measure the quality of care provided by nurses and rehabilitative therapists are managerial and educational. Managerial and educational support have been identified as crucial to the success of the initiative at every stage. For those starting at the beginning of the process it is important to identify sources of support in both these areas prior to initiating any form of the system. Finding one friendly, but influential, person is the key. If quality assurance is seen as positive, worthwhile and even enjoyable others will clamour to join in – at all levels of the organization. Starting in one area with all the back-up required and with staff who are enthusiastic and keen will prove to be infectious.

Practical issues

Once the support is established, the lines of communication drawn up, the initiative can begin. If adopting the system outlined in this manual, the Consensus Group will have identified the area of care to be addressed and will be ready to produce a standard of care. Take a standard from Part Two and adapt it and amend it until it suits the needs of the patient or client, the professional group that the Consensus Group represents and the health care environment in which care is provided. Then take an audit tool from Part Three and amend and adapt that until the questions suit the same needs that the standard had to be modified to address.

With the same Consensus Group work through the auditing guidelines determining the patient population, the timing and duration of the audit, how the questionnaires are to be completed and how the results of the audit are to be produced, and by whom. Ethical approval from the Ethics Committee within the health care organization may be necessary if patient opinion is to be sought as a part of the audit.

Once the results are available look at them carefully, decide whether additional information would be helpful to assist with interpretation, and then determine any plans for the implementation of any changes that are necessary – liaising with service and educational managers as appropriate. This is only the beginning of the process. It will evolve with the staff who use it and adapt it. But it is the beginning of a process that will assist with generating information which can be used in a variety of ways to achieve quality care.

Conclusion

This manual has been developed to be a practical guide to quality assurance. It is practical in the sense of defining the concept and the process of quality assurance, and the complex pressures and influences underlying that process. It is practical in the sense of providing the framework and examples of a system to put the process into action, and practical in addressing some of the many issues that arise from this activity.

Quality is described as subjective and elusive. This initiative to define and then measure quality in nursing and rehabilitative therapy demonstrates that this is not always the case. The implementation of change is a further issue and as Brook (1977) suggests:

'The central failing of quality assessment is that it has rarely been used to change behaviour and hence has not contributed much to the goal of improving health'.

If quality is to share equal status and equal weight in contracting for health services with cost-efficiency and cost-effectiveness, there must be evidence that changes occur and occur for the better. If change does not occur then quality will only ever be 'imperfectly achieved' (Brooks, 1989) and, as John Ruskin reflected with such accuracy, 'Quality is never an accident; it is always the result of intelligent effort'.

References

Audit Commission (1992) *Homeward Bound: A New Course for Community Health. Review.* HMSO, London.

Brook, R.J. (1977) Quality – can we measure it? *New England Journal of Medicine*, **296**, 170–72.

Brooks, T. (1989) *Best of Health: Winning Entries for the Hospital of the Year 1989.* Sunday Times/Andersen Consulting Health Care Practice, London.

Polit, D. & Hungler, B. (1987) *Nursing Research: Principles and Methods*, 3rd edn. J.B. Lippincott, Philadelphia.

PART TWO

STANDARDS OF CARE

Standards of Care

Chaplaincy

SPIRITUAL NEEDS

1. STANDARD STATEMENT

The aims of the chaplaincy for patients and their relatives who are experiencing spiritual distress are to facilitate and empower individuals in their search for meaning and purpose in life.

2. RATIONALE

All human beings have spiritual needs, which are often distinct from religious needs. These may be put into several categories:

(1) The need for meaning and purpose

(2) The need to love and be loved

(3) The need to forgive and be forgiven

(4) The need for hope and creativity   (Clinebell, 1976)

This is a complex experience that requires subtlety and sensitivity. The need for meaning and purpose is retrospective, the need to love and be loved is prospective, and the need to forgive and be forgiven and for hope and creativity deal with the present situation.

Spiritual needs become especially important for patients diagnosed as having cancer and their families. The perceived nature of the disease is that of one which is life threatening or curtailing, and focusses the attention of the individual and family on the transient nature of life.

Unfulfilled spiritual needs may lead to spiritual distress or pain. Although the problems of a whole lifetime may not be able to be addressed by the chaplains or other members of the multidisciplinary team, it is their role to offer support and care to patients and those caring for them while they attempt to attain or maintain spiritual integrity.

Rehabilitation enables patients to achieve their maximum quality of life, to be at one with themselves despite any limitations of the illness, and to be able to face with a degree of confidence whatever lies ahead. Spiritual rehabilitation does not lend itself early to a problem solving approach. Chaplaincy offers more pertinently affirmation of signs of spiritual health and a preparedness to be with people in distress. Equally important, chaplains provide support, education and consultancy to other members of the multi-disciplinary team facilitating their role in spiritual care.

3. RESOURCES

(1) A member of the chaplaincy team is available 24 hours a day.

(2) The chaplain will have a working knowledge of:

(a) The issues which often arise from the spiritual needs of the individual diagnosed with cancer.

(b) Signs and symptoms of altered spiritual integrity and their effect on interpersonal relationships.

(c) Strategies of coping with spiritual pain.

(d) Management of anticipatory and catastrophic grief.

(e) The pastoral/theological basis of responding to spiritual needs.

(f) The roles and skills of other members of the multidisciplinary team and the appropriateness of referrals.

(3) The chaplain will have skills in:

(a) Working as a member of a multi-faith, multi-cultural and multidisciplinary team.

(b) Communication: e.g. listening to patients and/or families review their lives, edifying patients who have lost their sense of hope.

(c) Teaching: e.g. for the education of other members of the multidisciplinary team in identifying and addressing spiritual needs.

(d) Being sensitive in action and word to differing belief systems and cultures.

(e) Applying pastoral and theological approaches in response to patient and families' spiritual needs.

(f) Providing liturgical forms which assist in the meeting of spiritual needs.

(4) The chaplain will have access to:

(a) Continuing education and information related to spiritual needs.

(b) Relevant multidisciplinary meetings.

(c) A system for documenting aspects of professional practice.

(d) Privacy and quiet whenever necessary for those requiring time, space and counsel.

(e) The time and resources to maintain his or her personal spiritual integrity.

(f) Suitable near-site accommodation.

(g) Current professional literature.

(h) Religious aids which may assist in meeting the spiritual needs of patients and families (e.g. relevant scriptures, holy pictures, prayer cards).

(i) An open referral system for patients, families, and staff.

4. PROFESSIONAL PRACTICE

(1) The chaplain makes an initial assessment of:

(a) The patient's perspective of his or her spiritual needs.

(b) Signs of impaired spiritual integrity and their effect on inter-personal relationships.

(c) Patient expectations of and desire for pastoral care.

(2) The chaplain offers care in co-operation with the patient, family, and other members of the multidisciplinary team.

(3) The chaplain provides a confidential service but, as negotiated with the patient and/or family, communicates appropriate information with the multidisciplinary team.

(4) Because of the uniqueness of spiritual needs to individuals, the chaplain uses an open approach which allows the patient to direct the encounter when appropriate.

(5) The chaplain maintains a lively consciousness of the uniqueness of each individual and provides care accordingly.

(6) If issues arise which would be better addressed by other disciplines, the chaplain refers to the appropriate health care professional.

(7) As issues arise, the chaplain may act as a resource to provide information and guidance to other members of the multidisciplinary team related to spiritual needs.

5. OUTCOMES

(1) The patient and/or family report that the chaplain's presence has been helpful and that they are satisfied with the pastoral care received.

(2) The chaplain reports that he or she had access to the resources needed and was able to follow professional practice. The chaplain will also report that the patient's spiritual needs were addressed and all possible steps were taken to restore integrity.

(3) Health care professionals will report that when they needed something from the chaplain related to the spiritual needs of patients, the chaplain responded quickly and offered enough information and education to allow the health care professional to address the problem should it arise again.

REFERENCES AND FURTHER READING

Cassel, E. J. (1982) The nature of suffering and the goals of medicine. New *England Journal Of Medicine*, **306 (2)**: 639–45.

Clinebell, H. J. (1976) *Basic Types of Counselling*. Abingdon, New York.

Eaton, G. (1985) *Islam and the Destiny of Man*. Islamic Texts Society Allen & Unwin, London.

Helman, C. G. (1990) *Culture, Health and Illness*. Wright, London.

Kushner, H. S. (1982) *When Bad Things Happen To Good People*. Pan Books, London.

McGilloway, O. and Myco, F. (1985) *Nursing and Spiritual Care*. Harper & Row, London.

Maddocks, M. (1991) *The Christian Healing Ministry*. SPCK, London.

Pattison, S. (1989) *Alive and Kicking: Towards a Practical Theology of Illness and Healing*. SCM Press, London.

Wald, F. S. (Ed) (1986) *In Quest of the Spiritual Component of Care for the Terminally Ill* (*Proceedings of a Colloquium*). Yale University Press, New Haven.

Standards of Care

Dietetic

GENERAL STANDARD OF ACCESS TO NUTRITIONAL SUPPORT FROM THE DIETETIC TEAM

1. STANDARD STATEMENT

Dietetic care for patients requiring nutritional support is directed towards enabling patients to achieve their optimum nutritional status.

2. RATIONALE

The ultimate undesired consequence of a compromised nutritional status is the occurrence of cachexia, a profound wasting syndrome characterized by weight loss, anorexia and muscle weakness. Cachexia can lead to malnutrition, infectious complications, poor well-being and ultimately death. The presence of malnutrition in cancer patients is associated with increased morbidity, decreased survival and decreased tolerance to cancer therapy. However, malnutrition should not be an obligatory response of the patient to cancer. There are now effective ways of maintaining and/or restoring nutritional status , and nutritional support should be considered as a major component of treatment in addition to anti-cancer therapy (Shils, 1979, Von Myenfeldt, 1988).

3. RESOURCES

(1) A State Registered dietitian is available to give advice, information and/or treatment.

(2) The dietitian will have a background knowledge of oncology and the effects of the disease and treatment upon the nutritional status of cancer patients. The dietitian should also have knowledge of the dietetic principles of care for such patients, including the use of enteral and parenteral feeding regimes.

(3) The dietitian will have skills to discuss these issues with the patient and family to gain their trust and co-operation and to offer encouragement and practical help with feeding difficulties or a particular diet.

(4) The dietitian will have access to educational and support programmes to ensure maintenance of the knowledge and skill base and to facilitate updated practice.

(5) Other members of the multidisciplinary team will be available to act as a source of referral or a resource to the patient, family and dietitian to facilitate continuity of care.

(6) The dietitian will have the co-operation of the catering department for practical assistance in the provision of appropriate food or particular diets.

(7) The dietitian will have available or access to, a range of practical equipment including:

- weighing scales
- microwave oven
- liquidizers and blenders
- substances for enteral feeding and general nutritional support
- delivery systems for these substances.

(8) The dietitian will have available written procedures related to enteral and parenteral feeding.

(9) The dietitian will have available written information for the patient and/or family (e.g. the patient information booklet *Overcoming Eating Difficulties* and diet sheets).

(10) The dietitian will have available a documentation system to record professional practice.

(11) The dietitian will have access to clerical help and office equipment including a telephone.

(12) There will be a referral system for other members of the multidisciplinary team to refer patients to the dietitian:

- New in-patient referrals will be seen by a dietitian within 48 hours of the referral. The exception to this is referrals made after 3.00 PM on Fridays which may not be seen until the Monday.
- Referrals for tube feeding or for specific therapeutic diets will be discussed with the medical team responsible before treatment commences.

(13) There will be a 'feedback' system to the referrer – verbal or written feedback will be given to the referring health care professional.

4. PROFESSIONAL PRACTICE

(1) The dietitian makes an initial and ongoing assessment of the patients' nutritional needs including information regarding:

- weight, past and present
- nutritional intake
- appetite changes
- biochemical parameters (if applicable)
- informational needs.

(2) The dietitian makes an initial and ongoing observation of the patient including information regarding:

- general appearance
- muscle weakness
- emaciation.

(3) The dietitian plans and implements interventions as a result of the assessment and in conjunction with the patient, family and other members of the multidisciplinary team.

(4) The dietitian offers the patient and family individualized information and teaching as appropriate.

(5) The dietitian evaluates and amends interventions as necessary as the ongoing assessment and/or observations dictate.

(6) The dietitian records all aspects of professional practice in departmental records and in the patient's care plan.

(7) The dietitian co-ordinates interventions with the members of the multidisciplinary team to facilitate an optimum level of care and attain and maintain continuity.

(8) The dietitian recommends nutritional interventions or refuses an aspect of care according to his or her professional expertise or code of conduct.

5. OUTCOMES

(1) The patient and family report that the nutritional needs of the patient were met at a practical level and at an informational/support level. They also report that they were satisfied with the care that they received.

(2) The dietitian considers that he or she had access to the resources as listed and was able to follow the described professional practice. The dietitian also reports that the patient achieve optimum nutritional status and that the nutritional needs of the patient were met at a practical level and at an informational/support level.

(3) The documentation system will show evidence that resources were used and professional practice followed in order that the patient could achieve optimum nutritional status. There will be evidence that the nutritional needs of the patient were met at a practical level and at an informational/support level.

REFERENCES

Shils, M. (1979) Principles of nutritional therapy. *Cancer*, **43**, 2093–102.
Von Myenfeldt, M. F. (1988) The aetiology and management of weight loss and malnutrition in cancer patients. *Baillière's Clinical Gastroenterology*, Vol 2, Part 4, 869–85.

NUTRITIONAL SUPPORT FOR CHILDREN

1. STANDARD STATEMENT

Dietetic care for children is directed towards achieving an optimum nutritional status and aims to enable children to enjoy their food.

2. RATIONALE

To many people the word 'cancer' is synonymous with malnutrition and eating difficulties. In children eating difficulties of particular significance include anorexia due to the disease, treatment or hospital admission, taste changes, mucositis, oesphagitis, dry mouth, nausea and vomiting and constipation.

Children who lose more than 10% of their ideal body weight risk having their treatment delayed or adapted, and this may ultimately affect its outcome. They may also experience poor wound healing and an increased susceptibility to infection (Van Eys, 1984, Rickard *et al.*, 1986).

Malnutrition is not an obligatory response to the host of cancer (Schils, 1979). However, for malnutrition to be prevented in children, it is essential that eating difficulties are identified and treated as they occur by specific dietary modification.

3. RESOURCES

(1) A state registered dietitian is available to give advice, information and/or treatment.

(2) The dietitian will have a background knowledge of oncology and the effects of the disease and treatment upon the nutritional status of children with cancer. The dietitian should also have knowledge of the dietetic principles of care for such patients including the use of enteral and parenteral feeding regimes.

(3) The dietitian will have specific skills to discuss these issues with the child and family to gain their trust and co-operation and to offer encouragement and practical help with feeding difficulties or a particular diet.

(4) The dietitian will have access to educational and support programmes to ensure maintenance of the knowledge and skill base and to facilitate updated practice.

(5) Other members of the multidisciplinary team will be available to act as a source of referral or a resource to the patient, family and dietitian to facilitate continuity of care.

(6) The dietitian will have the co-operation of the catering department for practical assistance in the provision of appropriate food or particular diets.

(7) The dietitian will have available, or have access to, a range of practical equipment including:

- weighing scales
- microwave oven
- liquidizers and blenders
- substances for enteral feeding and general nutritional support
- delivery systems for these substances.

DIETETIC

(8) An equipped kitchen will be available for the dietitian, ward staff and family/carers to enable them to prepare food at any time of the day.

(9) The dietitian will have available written procedures related to enteral and parenteral feeding.

(10) The dietitian will have access to written information specifically written or adapted for children.

(11) The dietitian will have available a documentation system to record professional practice.

(12) The dietitian will have access to clerical help and office equipment including a telephone.

(13) There will be a referral system for other members of the multidisciplinary team to refer patients to the dietitian.

- New in-patient referrals will be seen by a dietitian within 48 hours of the referral. The exception to this is referrals made after 3.00 PM on Fridays which may not be seen until the Monday.
- Referrals for tube feeding or for specific therapeutic diets will be discussed with the medical team responsible before treatment commences.

(14) There will be a 'feedback' system to the referrer – verbal or written feedback will be given to the referring health care professional.

4. PROFESSIONAL PRACTICE

(1) The dietitian makes an initial and ongoing assessment of the child's nutritional needs including information regarding:

- weight, past and present
- comparision of present weight and height with ideal weight and height for age using a growth and development record (Tanner & Whitehouse, 1975)
- nutritional intake
- appetite changes and their possible causes
- biochemical parameters (if applicable)
- informational needs of the child and family.

(2) The dietitian will make an initial and ongoing observation of the child including information regarding:

- general appearance
- muscle weakness
- emaciation.

(3) The dietitian plans and implements interventions as a result of the assessment and in conjunction with the child, family and other members of the multidisciplinary team.

(4) The dietitian offers the child and family individualized information and teaching as appropriate.

(5) The dietitian evaluates and amends interventions as necessary as the ongoing assessment and/or observations dictate.

(6) The dietitian records all aspects of professional practice in departmental records and in the child's care plan.

(7) The dietitian co-ordinates interventions with the members of the multidisciplinary team to facilitate an optimum level of care and attain and maintain continuity.

(8) The dietitian recommends nutritional interventions or refuses an aspect of care according to his or her professional expertise or code of conduct.

5. OUTCOMES

(1) The child and family report that the nutritional needs of the child were met at a practical level and at an informational/support level and that wherever possible the child enjoyed his or her food. They also report that they were satisfied with the care that they received.

(2) The dietitian considers that he or she had access to the resources as listed and was able to follow the described professional practice. The dietitian also reports that the child achieved optimum nutritional status, enjoyed his or her food, and that the nutritional needs of the child and family were met at a practical level and at an informational/ support level.

(3) The documentation system will show evidence that resources were used and professional practice followed in order for the child to achieve optimum nutritional status and to enjoy his or her food. There will be evidence that the nutritional needs of the child and family were met at a practical level and at an informational/support level.

REFERENCES

Rickard, K. A., Coates, J. D., Grosfield, J. L. *et al.* (1986) The value of nutritional support in children with cancer. *Cancer*, **58**, 1904–910.

Shils, M. (1979) Principles of nutritional therapy. *Cancer*, **43**, 2093–102.

Tanner, J. M. & Whitehouse, R. M. (1975) *Growth and Development Record*. Case wood Publications, Ware, Herts.

Van Eys, J. (1984) Nutrition in the treatment of cancer in children, *J. Am. Coll. Nutrition*, **3**, 159–68.

DIETETIC

NUTRITIONAL SUPPORT FOR IN-PATIENTS UNDERGOING CONTINUING CARE

1. STANDARD STATEMENT

Dietetic care for patients undergoing continuing care is directed towards achieving an optimum nutritional status. Nutritional support also aims to enable patients to enjoy their food and improve their quality of life.

2. RATIONALE

Nutritional support can play an important role in the care of patients with advanced cancer (Hunter & Janes, 1988). Anorexia, for example, is a frequent symptom experienced by up to 84% of continuing care patients (Gallagher, 1989). Care of patients with advanced disease concentrates on nutritional problems such as anorexia, nausea, and taste changes. Nutritional intervention may be of some benefit in controlling symptoms such as heartburn and constipation. Nutritional support may help to improve quality of life by avoiding the distress of excessive weight loss which can affect a patient's wellbeing (Shaw, 1989).

3. RESOURCES

(1) A state registered dietitian is available to give advice, information and/or treatment.

(2) The dietitian will have a background knowledge of oncology and the effects of the disease and treatment upon the nutritional status of patients with cancer. The dietitian should also have knowledge of the dietetic principles of care for such patients including the use of enteral and parenteral feeding regimes. The dietitian will be aware of the ethical considerations of feeding the terminally ill patient.

(3) The dietitian will also have a knowledge of feeding aids which may be necessary for physically debilitated people.

(4) The dietitian will have specific skills to discuss these issues with the patient and family to gain their trust and co-operation and to offer encouragement and practical help with feeding difficulties or a particular diet.

(5) The dietitian will have access to educational and support programmes to ensure maintenance of the knowledge and skill base and to facilitate updated practice.

(6) Other members of the multidisciplinary team will be available to act as a source of referral or a resource to the patient, family and dietitian to facilitate continuity of care.

(7) The dietitian will have the co-operation of the catering department for practical assistance in the provision of appropriate food or particular diets.

(8) The dietitian will have available, or have access to, a range of practical equipment including:

- weighing scales
- microwave oven
- liquidizers and blenders

- substances for enteral feeding and general nutritional support
- delivery systems for these substances.

(9) The dietitian will have available written procedures related to enteral and parenteral feeding.

(10) The dietitian will have available written information for the patient and/or family (e.g. the patient information booklet *Overcoming Eating Difficulties* and diet sheets).

(11) The dietitian will have available a documentation system to record professional practice.

(12) The dietitian will have access to clerical help and office equipment including a telephone.

(13) There will be a referral system for other members of the multidisciplinary team to refer patients to the dietitian:

- New in-patient referrals will be seen by a dietitian within 48 hours of the referral. The exception to this is referrals made after 3.00 PM on Fridays which may not be seen until the Monday.
- Referrals for tube feeding or for specific therapeutic diets will be discussed with the medical team responsible before treatment commences.

(14) There will be a 'feedback' system to the referrer; verbal or written feedback is given to the referring health care professional.

---

4. PROFESSIONAL PRACTICE

(1) The dietitian makes an initial and ongoing assessment of the patient's nutritional needs including information regarding:

- subjective changes in weight
- nutritional intake
- appetite changes
- informational needs.

(2) The dietitian plans and implements interventions as a result of the assessment, and in conjunction with the patient, family and other members of the multidisciplinary team.

(3) The dietitian offers the patient and family individualized information and teaching as appropriate.

(4) The dietitian evaluates and amends interventions as necessary as the ongoing assessment and/or observations dictate.

(5) When the patient is terminally ill, the dietitian – in collaboration with the patient, family and other members of the multidisciplinary team – discusses and adjusts the level of nutritional support accordingly.

(6) The dietitian records all aspects of professional practice in departmental records and in the patient's care plan.

(7) The dietitian co-ordinates interventions with the members of the multidisciplinary team to facilitate an optimum level of care and attain and maintain continuity.

(8) The dietitian recommends nutritional interventions or refuses an aspect of care according to his or her professional expertise or code of conduct.

5. OUTCOMES

(1) The patient and family report that the nutritional needs of the patient were met at a practical level and at an informational/support level. They also report that the patient was able to enjoy his or her food, and that they were satisfied with the care received.

(2) The dietitian considers that he or she had access to the resources as listed and was able to follow the described professional practice. The dietitian also reports that the patient achieved optimum nutritional status, was able to enjoy food, and that the nutritional needs of the patient were met at a practical level and at an informational/support level.

(3) The documentation system will show evidence that resources were used and professional practice followed in order for the patient to achieve optimum nutritional status. There will be evidence that the nutritional needs of the patient were met at a practical level and at an informational/support level, and that the patient was able to enjoy his or her food.

REFERENCES

Gallagher, C. (1989) *Nutritional Care for the Terminally Ill*, Chapter 9, Nutritional intervention and symptom control. Aspen Publications, Rockville, Maryland.

Hunter, M. and Janes, E. M. H. (1988) Nutrition in cancer care. In *Oncology for Nurses and Health Care Professionals*, (Ed. by R. Tiffany), pp. 138–64. Harper & Row, London.

Shaw, C. (1989) A taste of things to come. *Nursing Times*, **85(22)**, 26–8.

NUTRITIONAL SUPPORT FOR IN-PATIENTS UNDERGOING TREATMENT FOR HEAD AND NECK CANCERS

DIETETIC

1. STANDARD STATEMENT

Dietetic care for patients being treated for head and neck cancers is directed towards improving and/or maintaining their nutritional status during and after treatment.

2. RATIONALE

To many people, the word 'cancer' is synonymous with malnutrition. Progressive weight loss is the most obvious manifestation of neoplastic cachexia. Shils (1979) has pointed out that malnutrition is not an obligatory response to the host of cancer. Cancers of the head and neck often result in complex problems that may have a negative impact on the patient's nutritional status. Treatment may involve surgical excision, radical radiotherapy and/or chemotherapy – all of which have the potential for precipitating further nutritional problems. These problems are usually long term and therefore long term nutritional support is commonly required by these patients to maintain nutritional status, promote wound healing and to minimize the incidence and severity of complications of the various treatment modalities (Copeland *et al.*, 1979, Grant *et al.*, 1989).

3. RESOURCES

(1) A state registered dietitian is available to give advice, information and/or treatment.

(2) The dietitian will have a background knowledge of oncology and the effects of the disease and treatment upon the nutritional status of patients with cancer. The dietitian should also have knowledge of the dietetic principles of care for such patients including the use of enteral and parenteral feeding regimes.

(3) The dietitian will have skills to discuss these issues with the patient/family to gain their trust and co-operation and to offer encouragement and practical help with feeding difficulties or a particular diet.

(4) The dietitian will have access to educational and support programmes to ensure maintenance of the knowledge and skill base and to facilitate updated practice.

(5) Other members of the multidisciplinary team will be available to act as a source of referral or a resource to the patient, family and dietitian to facilitate continuity of care.

(6) The dietitian will have the co-operation of the catering department for practical assistance in the provision of appropriate food or particular diets.

(7) The dietitian will have available or have access to, a range of practical equipment including:

- weighing scales
- microwave oven
- liquidizers and blenders
- substances for enteral feeding and general nutritional support
- delivery systems for these substances.

(8) The dietitian will have available written procedures related to enteral and parenteral feeding.

(9) The dietitian will have available written information for the patient and/or family (e.g. the patient information booklet *Overcoming Eating Difficulties* and diet sheets).

(10) The dietitian will have available a documentation system to record professional practice.

(11) The dietitian will have access to clerical help and office equipment including a telephone.

(12) There will be a referral system for other members of the multidisciplinary team to refer patients to the dietitian.

- New in-patient referrals will be seen by a dietitian within 48 hours of the referral. The exception to this is referrals made after 3.00 PM on Fridays which may not be seen until the Monday.
- Referrals for tube feeding or for specific therapeutic diets will be discussed with the medical team responsible before treatment commences.

(13) There will be a 'feedback' system to the referrer; verbal or written feedback is given to the referring health care professional.

4. PROFESSIONAL PRACTICE

(1) The dietitian makes an initial and ongoing assessment of the patient's nutritional needs including information regarding:

- weight, past and present
- nutritional intake
- physical eating difficulties
- appetite changes
- biochemical parameters (if applicable)
- informational needs.

(2) The dietitian makes an initial and ongoing observation of the patient including information regarding:

- general appearance
- muscle weakness
- emaciation.

(3) The dietitian plans and implements interventions as a result of the assessment and in conjunction with the patient, family and other members of the multidisciplinary team.

(4) The dietitian offers the patient and family individualized information and teaching as appropriate.

(5) The dietitian evaluates and amends interventions as necessary, as the ongoing assessment and/or observations dictate.

(6) The dietitian liaises with the speech therapist with regard to swallowing difficulties and with the occupational therapist with regard to aids and/or equipment for eating.

(7) Patients are re-assessed by the dietitian on discharge and on subsequent out-patient visits.

(8) The dietitian records all aspects of professional practice in departmental records and in the patient's care plan.

(9) The dietitian co-ordinates interventions with the members of the multidisciplinary team to facilitate an optimum level of care and attain and maintain continuity.

(10) The dietitian recommends nutritional interventions or refuses an aspect of care according to his or her professional expertise or code of conduct.

5. OUTCOMES

(1) The patient and family report that the nutritional needs of the patient were met at a practical level and at an informational/support level. They also report that they were satisfied with the care received.

(2) The dietitian considers that he or she had access to the resources as listed and was able to follow the described professional practice. The dietitian also reports that the patient's nutritional status was maintained and/or improved during and after treatment and that the nutritional needs of the patient were met at a practical level and at an informational/support level.

(3) The documentation system will show evidence that resources were used and professional practice followed in order for the patient's nutritional status to be maintained and/or improved during and after treatment. There will be evidence that the nutritional needs of the patient were met at a practical level and at an informational/support level.

REFERENCES

Copeland, E. M., Daly, J. M. & Dudrick, S. J. (1979) Nutritional concepts of head and neck malignancies. *Head and Neck Surgery*, **March/April issue**, 350–63.

Grant, M., Rhiner, M. & Padilla, G. (1989) Nutritional management in the head and neck cancer patient. *Seminars in Oncology Nursing*, **5(3)**, 195–204.

Shils, M. (1979) Principles of nutritional therapy. *Cancer*, **43**, 2093–102.

Standards of Care

Nursing

CARE OF PATIENTS WHO MAY OR WHO ARE EXPERIENCING AN ALTERATION IN BODY IMAGE AS A RESULT OF BREAST CANCER AND/OR ITS TREATMENT

1. STANDARD STATEMENT

The nursing care for women who may or who are experiencing an alteration in body image as a result of breast cancer and/or its treatment is directed towards providing individualized practical advice, support and information enabling women to retain/regain their body image and to accept the changes in body image that have occurred.

2. RATIONALE

Schilder (1935) defined body image as 'the picture which we form in our mind, that is to say the way in which our body appears to ourselves'. This definition emphasizes a personal and subjective experience of the body.

Price (1990) describes a model of body image care based on certain key components. These include body reality (the body as it really exists), body ideal (the picture of our body in our heads depicting the way we should like to look and to perform), body presentation (the efforts made to match body reality to body ideal), coping strategies, social support network, environment and self-image. Self-image refers to the way in which we would describe ourselves, the kind of person we think we are (Gross, 1991). A healthy body image is considered to be an attribute that enhances self-image. Self-image, self-esteem or regard and ideal self form the basis of our self-concept.

Body image is said to be formed initially at pre-toddler stage and develops throughout life (Head, 1920). Each individual at some time encounters a potential or actual threat to this body image, and an alteration in body image may ensue. Women with breast cancer, for example, are exposed to the possibility of an alteration in body image at all stages of their disease and treatment. As Tait (1988) puts it, 'The female breast is regarded as the symbol of intrinsic femininity, sexual desirability and maternal comfort and succour. Breasts are central to many people's views about being a woman'. Consequently women undergoing breast surgery for example may experience severe problems related to body image (Maguire, 1978). A woman's response to actual or potential alterations in body image is influenced by a variety of factors including the availability of support from a partner and previous psychological problems (Denton & Baum, 1983). Counselling from the time of the diagnosis has been shown to help women cope with breast cancer (Watson *et al.*, 1988) and Fallowfield and colleagues (1986) suggest that this service should be provided for all women treated for breast cancer.

Nurses are in a unique position to assist patients and can be instrumental in enabling individuals to maintain and/or re-establish their body image. Nurses deal intimately with patients' hopes, fears and aspirations, and are advanced in the delivery of holistic care (Price, 1990). Price (1990) considers that following a body image assessment that incorporates actual and potential threats to each component of body image (i.e. body reality, body ideal, body presentation, coping strategies and social support networks), body image care can be categorized by five modes of typical care interventions. These are described as preventative care, supportive care, patient education, patient counselling and liaison with social support networks and other agencies. Evaluation of body image care by nurses is essential but needs to consider two important factors. Firstly, body image rehabilitation is frequently a long term process. Secondly evaluation can occur in one or more form – patient satisfaction with change, as well as nurses' observations of increased coping strategies, positive adjustment in body image and enhanced social support network (Price, 1990). Nurses therefore have a key role in the assessment, provision and evaluation of body image care for women with breast cancer.

3. RESOURCES

(1) The unit-based nurse will have a baseline knowledge of:

   (a) Theory and research on altered body image related to breast cancer and its treatment;
   (b) The psychological and social impact of altered body image;
   (c) The knowledge and skills of other health care professionals related to body image care;
   (d) The range of rehabilitative interventions;
   (e) Rehabilitative resources/services for referral;
   (f) Family dynamics and family functioning;
   (g) Issues related to sexuality and sexual functioning;
   (h) Physical and psychological consequences of treatment (all relevant modalities);
   (i) The impact of breast cancer and its treatment on work, social and leisure activities;
   (j) Management of lymphoedema;
   (k) Management of fungating wounds;
   (l) Prosthetics and clothing;
   (m) Reconstructive surgery.

(2) The unit-based nurse will have baseline skills in:

   (a) Communication (e.g. to provide information and support to the patient and family, to convey a sensitive and empathetic attitude and to assess the impact of altered body image);
   (b) Teaching (e.g. to offer the patient information and teaching about skin care);
   (c) Practical care (e.g. fitting of temporary prostheses).

(3) The unit-based nurse will have access to ongoing education and support. The clinical nurse specialist/unit manager will organize supervision, and unit-based teaching sessions, where necessary.

(4) The clinical nurse specialist (breast care) will have a detailed knowledge as listed in (1) – in particular the current trends and developments in breast care and the long term implications of breast cancer, its treatment and altered body image for the patient and family. The clinical nurse specialist (breast care) will also have a wider range of teaching and practical skills, and advanced communication skills, in order to assess the

initial impact of the diagnosis and/or the proposed treatment on the patient and to provide individualized information and support. The clinical nurse specialist (breast care) will also have skills related to the fitting of permanent prostheses. She or he will be available to act as a resource or source of referral for the patient, family and nurse.

(5) Other members of the multidisciplinary team who will be available to act as a resource or source of referral include the appliance officer, the physiotherapist, the social worker, the lymphoedema team, psychological care team and surgeons.

(6) There will be a range of specialist equipment available, e.g. prostheses, bras.

(7) Written information will be available to the patient and family. This will include radiotherapy and chemotherapy booklets, a hormonal therapy factsheet, hair loss booklet, information about bras, clothing and cosmetics, and information about reconstructive surgery.

(8) An environment suitable for the patient, family and nurse will be available – for example, a private and comfortable room for discussion and fitting of prostheses (including a full length mirror).

4. PROFESSIONAL PRACTICE

(1) The clinical nurse specialist (breast care) makes an initial assessment of the patient including the patient's family and support network, past experience of breast cancer and/or altered body image, feelings about treatment and its possible outcomes, the patient's feelings about herself and the features of the patient's appearance that are important to her. The clinical nurse specialist assesses the patient and family's level of knowledge and understanding and provides information and support tailored to their individual needs. The patient is followed up by the clinical nurse specialist throughout her hospital stay and on discharge. This may involve continued assessment of the impact of cancer and/or its treatment on the patient's body image, and self-image and self-esteem; and advice related to breast reconstruction.

(2) The unit-based nurse makes a pre-operative/pre-treatment assessment of:

   (a) The patient's home environment, the family structure and relationships, and the patient's level of emotional support;
   (b) The patient and family's feelings about the diagnosis, surgery and/or other treatment, and expectations related to altered body image and their priorities of concern.

(2) The unit-based nurse makes a post-operative/post-treatment assessment of:

   (a) Patient and family reactions to surgery/treatment;
   (b) Impact on family relationships and functioning (both immediate and long term);
   (c) Impact on self-image and on social and sexual functioning (both immediate and long term);
   (d) The patient's reaction to the physical appearance of the wound, skin, etc.
   (e) The patient and family's continued needs for information, support and education.

(3) The unit-based nurse plans and implements care in conjunction with the patient, family and other members of the multidisciplinary team:

(a) The patient and family are offered the opportunity to discuss concerns and express feelings related to altered body image;

(b) The nurse ensures wherever possible that the short and long term effects of disease and treatment to the breast are minimized (e.g. by offering instruction on skin care during radiotherapy, by providing symptomatic relief, etc.);

(c) For patients who have undergone surgery the nurse gently encourages the patient to look at the wound if appropriate, providing individualized and sensitive support;

(d) The nurse ensures that patients who have undergone breast surgery are offered a temporary prosthesis;

(e) The nurse offers the patient and family individualized information and support tailored to their individual and changing needs (e.g. related to self-esteem and feelings that the patient may experience, related to promoting self-image such as information about clothing, and information about support groups);

(f) The nurse liaises with the clinical nurse specialist (breast care) and discusses issues related to individual patient care.

(4) The unit-based nurse monitors and evaluates the effectiveness of care as in (1) and the appropriateness of interventions to meet individual needs.

(5) The unit-based nurse identifies the need to refer the patient to other members of the multidisciplinary team, will act where necessary as co-ordinator of the multidisciplinary team and will communicate appropriate information.

(6) The unit-based nurse facilitates continuity of care on discharge/transfer, consulting with the community liaison nurse where indicated and ensuring that the patient and/or family have a contact name or number for follow-up advice and support.

(7) The unit-based nurse documents accurately all aspects of professional practice.

5. OUTCOMES

(1) The patient and family feel that they received individualized practical advice, support and information; that they were able to retain/regain their body image and were moving towards accepting the changes that had occurred.

(2) The nurse considers that he or she had access to the resources as listed and was able to follow the described professional practice. The nurse also considers that the patient (and family) received individualized practical advice, support and information, and that the patient was able to retain/regain their body image and begin to accept the changes that had occurred.

(3) The documentation system will show evidence that resources were used and professional practice followed to ensure that the patient received individualized practical advice, support and information, that the patient was able to retain/regain his or her body image and is moving towards acceptance of the changes that occurred.

REFERENCES

Denton, S. & Baum, M. (1983) Psychological aspects of breast cancer. In *Contempory Issues in Clinical Oncology: Breast Cancer*, (Ed. by R. Margolese), pp. 173–85. Churchill Livingstone, Edinburgh.

Fallowfield, L. S., Baum, M. & Maguire, P. (1986) Effects of breast conservation on psychological morbidity associated with the diagnosis and treatment of early breast cancer. *British Medical Journal*, **293**, 1331–4.

Gross, R. D. (1991) *Psychology: The Science of Mind and Behaviour*. Hodder & Stoughton, London.

Head, H. (1920) *Studies in Neurology*. Oxford University Press, London.

Maguire, G. P., Lee, E. G., Bevington, D. J., Küchemann, C. S., Crabtree, R. J. & Connell, C. E. (1978) Psychiatric problems in the first year after mastectomy. *British Medical Journal*, **1**, 963–5.

Price, B. (1990) A model for body image care. *Journal of Advanced Nursing*, **15**, 585–93.

Tait, A. (1988) Whole or partial breast loss: the threat to womanhood. In *Altered Body Image*, (Ed. by M. Salter), pp. 167–78. John Wiley, Chichester.

Schilder, P. (1935) *The Image and Appearance of the Human Body*. Kegan Paul, London.

Watson, M., Denton, S., Baum, M. & Greer, S. (1988) Counselling breast cancer patients: a specialist nurse service. *Counselling Psychology Quarterly*, **1(1)**, 23–32.

NURSING

CARE OF PATIENTS EXPERIENCING ANOREXIA

NURSING

1. STANDARD STATEMENT

The nursing care of patients who may experience/are experiencing anorexia is directed towards maintaining an adequate nutritional status and the minimization of complications. The patient and family will be offered individualized information and support.

2. RATIONALE

Anorexia is a frequent and often demanding symptom in patients with cancer (De Wys, 1979) and is defined as a decreased appetite associated with a decrease in spontaneous food intake (Behnke, 1986). Patients complain of a loss of appetite and a tendency to feel 'full' after ingesting only a small amount of food. Appetite may be defined as that set of signals which guide the selection and consumption of specific foods and nutrients (Castonguay et al., 1983). Anorexia occurs therefore when these signals are absent or abnormal for any reason, causing the individual to lose the desire for food.

There are many physiological factors which cause anorexia including toxic effects of chemotherapy, anorexigenic substances secreted by tumour cells (Wesdorf & Krause, 1983), distressing symptoms, early satiety, taste and smell changes and oral-gustatory problems (Berstein, 1986) as well as psychological and sociocultural factors. The consequences of anorexia for the patient can include weight loss, prolonged healing time and fatigue. Therefore, the successful management of anorexia requires a careful and considered evaluation of the patient as a whole, taking into consideration whether the anorexia is likely to be a long or short term problem. Nursing care in conjunction with dietetic colleagues focusses on maintaining an adequate nutritional status wherever possible and minimizing the complications of anorexia.

3. RESOURCES

(1) The unit-based nurse will have a baseline knowledge of:

(a) The anatomy and physiology of the gastrointestinal tract;

(b) The potential effects of cancer and/or its treatment on the gastrointestinal tract;

(c) Nutritional assessment and nutritional requirements for adults;

(d) When to refer the patient to the dietitian;

(e) The possible causes of anorexia, including side-effects of treatment, effects of disease and psychological distress;

(f) The agents available to minimize the effects of cancer and/or its treatment on appetite (e.g. anti-emetics, anti-fungals etc.);

(g) Non-pharmacological methods of increasing appetite (e.g. offering small meals, liquid high calorie supplements, fortifying food and drinks, liquid meal replacements etc.);

(h) The indications for the initiation of either enteral or parenteral feeding;

(i) The potential effects of poor nutritional intake due to anorexia (e.g. weight loss, prolonged healing time, weakness and lethargy etc.);

(j) The potential psychological and social impact of anorexia for the patient and family.

(2) The unit-based nurse will have baseline skills in:

(a) Communication (e.g. listening skills and awareness of non-verbal cues to assess the psychological and social status of the patient; skills in conveying an empathetic and supportive attitude);

(b) Teaching to educate the patient and family about the causes of anorexia and, in conjunction with the dietitian, to offer advice on how to adapt while in hospital and on return home (e.g. bringing in food from home if appropriate, using high calorie supplements);

(c) Practical techniques (e.g. in oral care, drug administration and administration of nutritional supplements both enterally and parenterally, and the use and preparation of all ward-based dietary supplements).

(3) The unit-based nurse will have access to on-going education and support. The clinical nurse specialist/unit manager will organize supervision, and unit-based teaching sessions, where necessary.

(4) The clinical nurse specialist/unit manager is expected to have detailed knowledge as listed in (1) and skills as in (2).

(5) Other members of the multidisciplinary team will be available to act as a resource or source of referral to the patient, family and nurse including dietitians, social workers, occupational therapists, pharmacists, catering manager, oral hygienist and members of the patient's medical team.

(6) A range of well maintained and effective equipment is available on the ward, including:

- microwave oven
- fridge/freezer
- kettle
- toaster
- cooker
- liquidizer/blender
- basic foodstuffs
- supply of basic cutlery and crockery
- substances for enteral feeding and general nutritional support
- delivery systems for these substances.

(7) Written information will be available to the patient and family, including patient information booklets on eating difficulties, differing cancers and chemotherapy.

(8) Written information will be available to nurses on the ward including the chemotherapy protocols and information about side-effects.

(9) An environment suitable to the needs of the patient and family will be available, including a comfortable area for patients to have their meals.

(10) An environment to meet the needs/requirements of the nurse will be available including space and facilities to allow both hot and cold meals to be served attractively.

4. PROFESSIONAL PRACTICE

(1) The unit-based nurse makes an initial and ongoing assessment of:

(a) The patient's dietary history, including pre-illness appetite, food preferences, etc.;

(b) Changes in the patient's appetite and dietary intake since becoming ill and/or commencing treatment;

(c) The patient's physical appearance – for example, obvious signs of weight loss/malnutrition, etc. and the condition of the patient's mouth;

(d) The patient's current weight and percentage weight change since becoming ill;

(e) The potential complications arising from anorexia;

(f) The potential effects of planned treatment on the patient's nutritional status;

(g) Symptoms which may be causing anorexia – for example, taste and smell changes, stomatitis, pain, etc.;

(h) Psychological factors contributing to anorexia, such as low mood or anxiety;

(i) The psychological and social effects of anorexia on the patient and family;

(j) The educational needs of the patient and family concerning the patient's nutritional needs and the problem of anorexia;

(k) The patient's home environment and the support available to the patient following discharge, (e.g. to buy and prepare food), the dietary supplements available on prescription;

(l) The need to refer the patient to the dietitian.

(2) The unit-based nurse plans and implements care in conjunction with the patient, family and other relevant members of the multidisciplinary team.

(a) The patient and family are offered information about anorexia and advice on how to overcome/cope with it (including written information booklets).

(b) The patient is helped to choose appropriate foods from the menu and the family are encouraged to bring in food from home (where appropriate).

(c) The nurse administers prescribed pharmacological agents to reduce/prevent the symptoms causing anorexia (e.g. anti-emetics, analgesics, etc.), and liaises with medical colleagues to ensure optimum symptom control.

(d) Where appropriate, the nurse administers pharmacological/non-pharmacological agents to increase appetite (e.g. steroids, sherry, etc.)

(e) The patient is offered high calorie dietary supplements or is fed enterally or parenterally (where necessary).

(f) Where indicated, the nurse refers the patient to the dietitian and liaises with the dietitian, pharmacist and medical staff to ensure optimum nutritional support.

(g) The nurse provides nutritional support as requested/instructed by the dietitian.

(h) The patient and family are offered psychological support in coping with the problem of anorexia.

(i) The patient is offered education about oral hygiene.

(j) The nurse, in collaboration with the dietitian, provides the patient with information related to the management of anorexia when the patient is at home.

(3) The unit-based nurse monitors and evaluates the effectiveness of care as in (1) and the appropriateness of interventions to meet individual needs.

(4) The unit-based nurse will identify the need to refer the patient to other members of the multidisciplinary team where appropriate, will act where necessary as co-ordinator of the multidisciplinary team and will communicate appropriate information.

(5) The unit-based nurse will facilitate continuity of care following discharge/transfer consulting with the community liaison nurse where indicated and ensuring that the patient and/or family have a contact name and number for follow-up advice and information.

(6) The unit-based nurse documents accurately all aspects of professional practice.

5. OUTCOMES

(1) The patient and family report that the patient felt able to cope with anorexia and that complications were minimized. They also feel that their needs for education and for practical and emotional support were met.

(2) The nurse considers that he or she had access to the resources as listed and was able to follow the described professional practice. The nurse also felt able to meet the needs of the patient and family by providing optimal nutritional support and by minimizing both the causes and complications of anorexia.

(3) The documentation will show evidence that resources were used and professional practice followed resulting in maintenance or improvement of the patient's nutritional status and the minimization of complications. There will also be evidence that the patient and family's needs for education and for practical and emotional support were met.

REFERENCES

Behnke, M. C. (1986) Anorexia. In *Pathophysiological Phenomena in Nursing*, (Ed. by V. K. Camere, A. M. Lindsey and C. M. West), pp. 99–121. Saunders, Philadelphia.

Berstein, I. L. (1986) Etiology of anorexia in cancer. *Cancer*, **58**, 1881–6.

Castonguay, T. W., Applegate, E. A., Upton, D. E., & Stern, T. S. (1983) Hunger and appetite: old concepts, new distinctions. *Nutrition Reviews*, **41**, 101–110.

De Wys, W. D. (1979) Anorexia as a general effect of cancer. *Cancer*, **43**, 2013–19.

Wesdorp, R. L., Krause, R., & von-Meyenfeldt, M. F. (1983) Cancer cachexia and its nutritional its implications. *British Journal of Surgery*, **70(6)**, 352–5.

CARE OF PATIENTS EXPERIENCING ANXIETY

1. STANDARD STATEMENT

Nursing care is directed towards accurate assessment of anxiety. Patients will be offered practical help, support and/or information to prevent and/or reduce the distressing effects of anxiety.

2. RATIONALE

The experience of anxiety is highly personal and can be affected by past feelings and situations. The feeling of anxiety as it relates to cancer is no exception (Degoratis *et al.*, 1983, McCorkle *et al.*, 1983). Welch-McCaffrey (1985) describes anxiety as the 'escalated and frequently disruptive tension associated with uneasy feeling of potential harm and distress'. In addition, an array of signs and symptoms are usually associated with these uneasy feelings including nausea, anorexia, diarrhoea and vomiting (Rosenbaum, 1982). These are at times difficult to distinguish from the effects of cancer and/or treatment.

The impact of cancer is traumatic and stressful and often evokes a particularly intense emotional response (Sutherland, 1981). Anxiety is a natural response to threatening situations and is therefore a common but not universal component of patients' experience (Gobel & Donovan, 1987). The causes of cancer related anxiety have been carefully considered by Weisman (1979) who was able to delineate seven major areas including health, self-appraisal, work and finances, religion, family and significant relationships, friends and associates and existential concerns.

The psychological morbidity associated with cancer and its treatment has been well documented. During the late 1970s, studies looking at the rehabilitation needs of cancer patients identified anxiety and depression as common problems (Donovan, 1986). More recently however the universality of the association of anxiety, depression and hostility, and a diagnosis of cancer have been openly challenged with several authors reporting low incidence of psychological symptoms (e.g. McCorkle *et al.*, 1983, Cassileth *et al.*, 1984). For a significant minority of patients however anxiety can be so severe and/or persistent as to interfere with their daily lives and their ability to function.

The literature has also highlighted a discrepancy between what health care professionals perceived were the emotional responses of their patients and the patients' own perceptions (Derogatis *et al.*, 1979). While Maguire (1985) reported that the psychological problems of cancer were overlooked by health care professionals; psychological symptoms were not systematically assessed but their existence or absence assumed. Nurses have a key role in the assessment of patients' psychological needs and the individualization of care through a holistic multidisciplinary approach. Nurses can also implement measures which have been shown to prevent (and/or relieve) anxiety in particular, giving information and teaching (e.g. Hayward, 1975).

3. RESOURCES

(1) The unit-based nurse will have a baseline knowledge of the following.

    (a) The information required to make a comprehensive assessment of the actual presence of anxiety, including:

        ● the physical signs of anxiety (e.g. palpitations, tremor, sweating, dry mouth, anorexia and weight loss, sleep disturbance) and how these may be differentiated from symptoms which are a direct result of the disease processes

NURSING

- the emotional and behaviourial signs of anxiety (e.g. tension, agitation, irritability, poor concentration), and how to recognize them.

(b) The possible investigations and treatments for cancer and their adverse effects.

(c) The potential impact of cancer and its treatment as stressors, and anxiety as a response to these.

(d) The potential physical effects of anxiety on the patient and family (e.g. slower recovery from surgery, greater risk of post-operative complications).

(e) The potential impact of anxiety on psychological behaviour (e.g. disrupted family relationships, difficulty in assimilating and retaining information.

(f) The methods of alleviating anxiety.

(g) When it is appropriate to refer the patient and/or family for specialist help (e.g. to the psychological care team), and how to utilize the referral system.

(2) The unit-based nurse will have baseline skills in:

(a) Communication – for example, listening and observational skills to enable correct identification of patients and relatives who are/may become anxious, and skills to provide support which may prevent/reduce the effects of anxiety.

(b) Teaching – for effective education of the patient and family as to the possible effects of anxiety and methods of relieving these effects (e.g. relaxation, diversional therapy, etc.)

(c) Practical techniques – for example, in assessing physical signs of anxiety and in the use of methods to relieve anxiety.

(3) The unit-based nurse will have access to ongoing education and support. The clinical nurse specialist/unit manager will organize supervision, and unit-based teaching sessions, where necessary.

(4) The clinical nurse specialist/unit manager is expected to have detailed knowledge as listed in (1) and skills as in (2). Where the problem has specific management issues/ difficulties, a clinical nurse specialist/unit manager with specialist knowledge and skills may be identified to act as a consultant for advice and support.

(5) Other members of the multidisciplinary team will be available to act as a resource or source of referral to the patient, family and nurse including the psychological care team, chaplains, social workers, art therapist, therapeutic masseur and medical staff.

(6) There will be a range of information booklets available for patients and their families about cancer in general and the treatment of cancer.

(7) Information about the services/support groups available to cancer patients outside the hospital (e.g. CancerLink, BACUP) will be available to the nurse, patient and family.

(8) An environment acceptable to the patient and family will be available wherever possible – for example a private, comfortable interview room, free access for visitors, separate sitting room, etc.

(9) An environment suitable for the nurse to be able to assess the patient's and/or family's anxiety (e.g. access to a room for patient/nurse consultation) will be available.

4. PROFESSIONAL PRACTICE

(1) The unit-based nurse makes an initial assessment of the following.

(a) Previous history of anxiety and/or depression including any history of previous psychological problems.
(b) Previous experience of cancer (e.g. a friend or family member with cancer, media influence).
(c) The patient and family's response to previous stressful events and previous coping strategies employed.

(2) The unit-based nurse makes an initial and ongoing assessment of the following.

(a) The response of the patient and family to the present illness, their understanding of its implications and any current concerns.
(b) The patient and family's needs for support, information and teaching.
(c) Physical signs of anxiety.
(d) Emotional and behavioral signs of anxiety including the use of recognizable defence mechanisms (e.g. denial, regression, etc.)
(e) Any non-illness factors which may be contributing to or exacerbating anxiety, (e.g. marital difficulties, financial problems, etc.) and the need to refer for specialist help (e.g. to social worker)
(f) The availability of social support and other factors which mitigate the effects of stress.

(3) The unit-based nurse plans and implements care in conjunction with the patient, family, clinician and other members of the multidisciplinary team.

(a) The nurse offers individualized information and teaching.
(b) Where appropriate, the nurse enables the patient and family to understand their anxiety as a common response to the present situation.
(c) The patient and family are offered practical help, support and information related to the relief of anxiety (e.g. offering appropriate supportive therapy, giving clear written information, offering time to discuss anxieties, etc.)
(d) The nurse offers psychological care to the patient experiencing anxiety and to the patient's family.
(e) The nurse administers prescribed pharmacological therapies for the relief of anxiety (where appropriate).
(f) The nurse consults with other health care professionals about the management of anxiety and where necessary refers the patient for specialist care.

(4) The unit-based nurse monitors and evaluates the effectiveness of care as in (1) and the appropriateness of interventions to meet individual needs.

(5) The unit-based nurse will identify the need to refer the patient to other members of the multidisciplinary team where appropriate, will act where necessary as co-ordinator of the multidisciplinary team and will communicate appropriate information.

(6) The unit-based nurse will facilitate continuity of care following discharge/transfer, consulting with the community liaison nurse where indicated. Prior to discharge the nurse ensures that the patient and/or family have a contact name and number for follow-up advice and information.

NURSING

(7) The unit-based nurse documents accurately all aspects of professional practice.

5. OUTCOMES

(1) The patient and family report that they were provided with appropriate practical help, support and/or information to alleviate their anxiety.

(2) The nurse considers that he or she had access to the resources as listed and was able to follow the described professional practice. The nurse also reports that patients and their families who were experiencing anxiety were provided with appropriate practical help, support and/or information to alleviate their anxiety.

(3) The documentation system will show evidence that resources were used and professional practice followed to ensure that patients and their families who were experiencing anxiety were provided with appropriate practical help, support and/or information to alleviate their anxiety.

REFERENCES

Cassileth, B. R., Lusk, E. J., Strouse, T. B. *et al.* (1984) Psychosocial status in chronic illness. *New England Journal of Medicine*, **311**, 506–11.

Derogatis, L. R., Abeloff, M. D. & McBeth, C. D. (1979) Cancer patients and their physicians in the perception of psychological symptoms. *Psychomatics*, **17**, 197–201.

Derogotis, L. R., Marrow, G. R., Felting, J. *et al.* (1983) The prevelance of psychiatric disorders among cancer patients. *Journal of the American Medical Association*, **249**, 751–7.

Donovan, M. (1986) Symptom management – The nurse is the key. In *Issues and Topics in Cancer Nursing*, (Ed. by R. McCorkle & G. Hongaladarom), pp. 125–37. Appleton-Century-Crofts, Newark, CT.

Gobel, B.H. & Donovan M.I. (1978) Depression and anxiety. *Seminars in Oncology Nursing*, **3(4)**, 267–76.

Hayward, J. (1975) *Information – A Prescription Against Pain*. Royal College of Nursing, London.

McCorkle, R. & Quint-Benoliel, J. (1983) Symptom distress, current concerns, and mood disturbance after diagnosis of life threatening disease. *Social Science and Medicine*, **17**, 431–8.

Maguire, P. (1985) Improving the detection of psychiatric problems in cancer patients. *Social Science and Medicine*, **20**, 819–23.

Rosenbaum, J. F. (1982) Current concepts in psychiatry – the drug treatment of anxiety. *Medical Intelligence*, **306**, 401–4.

Sutherland, A. M. (1981) The psychological impact of cancer and its therapy. **31(3)**, 159–70.

Weisman, A. D. (1979) *Coping with Cancer*. McGraw-Hill, New York.

Welch-McCaffrey, D. (1985) Cancer, anxiety and quality of life. *Cancer Nursing*, **8**, 151–8.

CARE OF PATIENTS WITH ASCITES

1. STANDARD STATEMENT

The nursing care of patients with ascites is directed towards the promotion of safety and comfort through the relief or minimization of symptoms and the prevention/control of the complications associated with ascites. The patient and family will be offered comprehensive information and psychological support in order to help them cope with and adapt to this chronic problem.

2. RATIONALE

Malignant peritoneal effusion is a common and distressing symptom associated with carcinoma of the ovary, endometrium and breast. Several factors may contribute to the development of ascites, but the most common cause is peritoneal seeding from a tumour causing obstruction of diaphragmatic lymphatics (Zehner & Hoogstraten, 1985).

The symptoms which may result from ascites include loss of appetite, indigestion, weight gain, enlarging waist, dyspnoea, orthopnoea, constipation (caused by decreased bowel motility), nausea and vomiting and general discomfort. Nurses are responsible for assessing these symptoms and their effect(s) on the patient and family.

Nursing management of ascites focusses on patient comfort and safety — i.e. on the prevention of complications associated with ascites and with the drainage of ascitic fluid, and on patient and family education and support. Ascites, although presenting early, is more often a symptom of advanced cancer. It tends, therefore, to be an indication of either relapse or failure to respond to treatment. In view of this, psychological support is essential. Nurses play a key role in co-ordinating a multidisciplinary approach to care in order to facilitate the promotion of safety and patient comfort.

3. RESOURCES

(1) The unit-based nurse will have a baseline knowledge of the following.

   (a) The anatomy and physiology related to the development of ascites.
   (b) Possible causes of ascites.
   (c) Diagnostic tests used in the management of ascites (e.g. ultrasound).
   (d) Symptoms commonly associated with ascites (e.g. fatigue, breathlessness, discomfort/pain and constipation) and how they may be relieved.
   (e) Potential complications of ascites (e.g. bowel obstruction, electrolyte imbalance and nutritional deficits) and how to prevent, recognize and manage these.
   (f) The psychological impact of ascites on the patient and family specifically related to altered body image and the chronic nature of the problem.
   (g) The possible effects of the ascites on personal and sexual relationships, social activities and work activities.
   (h) Nursing care related to the drainage of ascitic fluid, including care of catheter and site, and the potential complications of catheter insertion (e.g. bowel perforation, shock etc.)
   (i) Current research and trends in the management of ascites, and their implications for the patient and family as well as for related nursing care.

(2) The unit-based nurse will have baseline skills in the following.

   (a) Communication — to convey a sensitive and empathetic attitude in order to gain the confidence of the patient and family, and to provide individualized support.

NURSING

    (b) Teaching – to provide information to the patient and family as to the cause(s) of ascites, its associated symptoms and management.

    (c) Practical techniques – for example to assist with catheter insertion, in care of catheter and catheter site.

(3) The unit-based nurse will have access to ongoing education and support. The clinical nurse specialist/unit manager will organize supervision, and unit-based teaching sessions, where necessary.

(4) The clinical nurse specialist/unit manager is expected to have detailed knowledge as listed in (1) and skills as in (2). Where the problem has specific management issues/difficulties or has become persistent and intractable a clinical nurse specialist/unit manager with specialist knowledge and skills may be identified to act as a consultant for advice and support.

(5) Other members of the multidisciplinary team will be available to act as a source of referral or a resource to the patient, family and nurse, including dietitians and medical staff.

(6) There will be a range of specialist equipment and therapeutic agents available for the management of ascites, including an adequate supply of equipment for catheter insertion and drainage.

(7) A range of written information on issues related to the patient's illness will be available to the patient and family. These may include information booklets on chemotherapy and ovarian cancer, as well as details of the relevant support services.

(8) Written information on the care of patients undergoing drainage of ascites will be available to the nurse on the ward (see *The Royal Marsden Hospital Manual of Clinical Procedures* Chapter 1, pp. 1–4).

(9) An environment suitable to the patient's individual needs will be available, for example privacy will be ensured where appropriate.

(10) An environment to meet the needs/requirements of the nurse (e.g. clean area to prepare trolley for aseptic procedures will be available).

4. PROFESSIONAL PRACTICE

(1) The unit-based nurse makes an initial and ongoing assessment of the following.

    (a) Symptoms associated with the ascites (e.g. pain, breathlessness, fatigue).

    (b) The stage of the patient's illness and treatment.

    (c) Any previous and/or current treatment and its effects on the patient.

    (d) The patient's weight and girth measurement (where appropriate).

    (e) The patient's nutritional status and dietary intake.

    (f) Previous history of ascitic drainage and associated problems.

    (g) The psychological response of the patient and family to the present admission, the problem of ascites and its short and long term implications.

    (h) The informational needs of the patient and family concerning the nature of ascites (e.g. its causes, symptoms and management), and the short and long term implications.

    (i) The effects of the ascites on the personal relationships, social activities and work activities of the patient.

(2) When the insertion of a drainage catheter is indicated the unit-based nurse makes a further assessment of:

(a) The amount, colour and consistency of the drainage.
(b) Signs of systemic infection as well as local infection around the drain site.
(c) Signs of any complication (e.g. shock, bowel perforation).

(3) The unit-based nurse plans and implements care in conjunction with the patient, family, and other members of the multidisciplinary team.

(a) Where the patient is experiencing symptoms such as pain or constipation, the nurse administers pharmacological and non-pharmacological interventions directed towards symptom relief, and liaises with medical colleagues where appropriate.
(b) Where the patient is experiencing fatigue and/or breathlessness the nurse assists with activities of daily living (according to the wishes of the individual) and offers to teach the patient methods to conserve energy and rest.
(c) When the insertion of a drainage catheter is indicated the nurse:

- prepares the patient and family for the procedure, offering individualized information and psychological support
- assists with and cares for the patient following the procedure according to *The Royal Marsden Hospital Manual of Clinical Nursing Procedures* Chapter 1, pp. 1–4.

(d) The nurse advises the patient and family on suitable clothing (e.g. cotton fabrics, clothes with loose or no waistband).
(e) The patient and family are offered information and psychological care according to their individual and changing needs.

(4) The unit-based nurse monitors and evaluates the effectiveness of care as in (1) and the appropriateness of interventions to meet individual needs.

(5) The unit-based nurse will identify the need to refer the patient to other members of the multidisciplinary team where appropriate, will act where necessary as co-ordinator of the multidisciplinary team and will communicate appropriate information.

(6) The unit-based nurse will facilitate continuity of care following discharge/transfer consulting with the community liaison nurse where indicated. Prior to discharge the nurse ensures that the patient and/or family have a contact name and number for follow-up advice and information.

(7) The unit-based nurse documents accurately all aspects of professional practice.

5. OUTCOMES

(1) The patient and family report that the symptoms associated with the ascites were relieved or minimized. They also feel that their needs for education and for practical and emotional support were met.

(2) The nurse considers that he or she had access to the resources as listed and was able to follow the described professional practice. The nurse also considers that he or she was able to meet the needs of the patient and family by relieving or minimizing symptoms, by preventing or controlling the complications of ascites and by offering information and support.

NURSING

(3) The documentation system will show evidence that resources were used and professional practice followed to ensure that patients' symptoms associated with their ascites were relieved or minimized, and complications prevented or controlled. There will also be evidence that the patient and family's needs for education and for practical and emotional support were met.

REFERENCE

Zehner, L. C. & Hoogstraten, B. (1985) Malignant effusions and their management. *Seminars in Oncology Nursing*, **1(4)**, 259–68.

CARE OF PATIENTS WITH A CENTRAL VENOUS LINE

1. STANDARD STATEMENT

The nursing care of patients with a central venous line is directed towards maintaining catheter patency, and the prevention, early detection and minimization of complications. Nursing care is also directed towards ensuring that the patient and/or family are competent and feel confident in the care of the central venous line. The patient and family will be offered comprehensive information, education and support.

2. RATIONALE

Patients with cancer often require intravenous therapy over a long period of time. Insertion of a central venous catheter will enable them to receive chemotherapy and support treatments such as total parentral nutrition (TPN), blood products, fluids and other intravenous medications without multiple venepuncture. The central venous catheter can also be used to obtain blood specimens for diagnostic purposes and for central venous pressure monitoring.

The central venous catheter is usually made from silicone rubber and is inserted under local or general anaesthetic into a main blood vessel. As it is inert, irritation to the vein is minimized allowing the catheter to remain in position for long periods. The central venous catheter is available with single, double and triple lumen that provide multiple access. The nature of the catheter facilitates freedom of movement and it can be concealed under clothing, which can enhance a person's quality of life. For some, it can provide reassurance that treatment is being undertaken.

The potential complications of a line include infection (particularly in those who become neutropenic), air embolism, blockage of the line, severing of the line and cracking of the hub. Patients may find their body image altered by the presence of the catheter, which can also be a constant reminder of the fact that they have cancer.

The role of the nurse is to ensure that problems are minimized in order to allow patients to continue their normal activities wherever possible, while ensuring the patency of catheters is maintained. Minimal handling of catheters and good aseptic technique reduces the risk of infection for example. Continuing education and support of patients and their family are essential to enable patients to be independent and retain a degree of control. Nurses have a responsibility to ensure that patients and/or other family members feel confident and competent in the care of the line, and that wherever possible the line remains functional.

3. RESOURCES

(1) The unit-based nurse will have a baseline knowledge of the following:

   (a) The nature of a central venous line and its indications for use.
   (b) The potential complications of the central venous line (e.g. superior vena cava obstruction, thrombosis and infection) and the signs and symptoms of these complications.
   (c) The surgical procedure for the insertion of the central venous line and whether this is carried out under general or local anaesthetic.
   (d) The principles of asepsis.
   (e) The day-to-day management of the line, and the insertion and exit sites.
   (f) The management of emergencies such as cut or cracked lines, exposure of the cuff, damaged ends of line and extravasation.
   (g) The psychological implications of a central venous line for a patient (e.g. the line

as a constant reminder of the patient's illness, feelings related to altered body image etc.)

(h) The implications of a central venous line on the patient's work, social and leisure activities.

(i) Current research and trends in the management of central venous lines and their implications for both the patient and family and related nursing care.

(2) The unit-based nurse will have baseline skills in:

(a) Communication – to convey a confident, competent and empathetic attitude and to provide individualized information and support. Also observational skills to assess the line.

(b) Teaching – to demonstrate and educate the patient and family in the care of the line and to ensure they are aware of potential complications.

(c) Practical techniques (e.g. possession of the Drug Administration Certificate and skills related to the care of the line and the management of potential complications).

(3) The unit-based nurse will have access to ongoing education and support. The clinical nurse specialist/unit manager will organize supervision, and unit-based teaching sessions, where necessary.

(4) The intravenous services clinical nurse specialist/unit manager will have detailed knowledge and skills as listed in (1) and (2). She or he will provide expert nursing care to patients with persistent or unusual complications with the catheter (e.g. blocked lines, extravasations) and to patients requiring complicated intravenous systems to receive their chemotherapy. She or he will also supervise care to ensure that closed systems are maintained, systems correctly matched to patients, and patient education provided to ensure the safety of individuals with tunnelled catheters.

(5) Other members of the multidisciplinary team will be available to act as a resource or source of referral to the patient, family and nurse including clinical nurse specialist (infection control), medical staff and pharmacists.

(6) There will be a range of basic equipment available to the patient, family and nurse including IV packs, trolleys/trays, central venous line repair kits, luer lock equipment and equipment for the disposal of sharps.

(7) The nurse will have access to current written information and research, including chemotherapy protocols, and *The Royal Marsden Hospital Manual of Clinical Nursing Procedures* (Chapter 9, pp. 109–130).

(8) Written information will be available to the patient and family including teaching packages on care of a central venous line.

(9) An environment suitable to the patient's individual needs will be available including, for example, access to privacy for information giving, teaching and support.

(10) An environment to met the needs/requirements of the nurse (e.g. a clean area to prepare equipment) will be available.

4. PROFESSIONAL PRACTICE

(1) The unit-based nurse makes an initial and ongoing assessment of:

  (a) The reason for the insertion of a central venous line.
  (b) The patient and family's knowledge and previous experience of central venous lines.
  (c) The patient and family's ability (e.g. their visual acuity and manual dexterity) and willingness to participate in the management and care of the line.
  (d) The patient's general physical condition (e.g. their level of mobility, condition of skin).
  (e) The patient's psychological status (e.g. whether the patient is anxious, confused or experiencing short term memory loss).
  (f) Whether the patient and/or family experience comprehension difficulties (e.g. perceptual problems/language problems) and whether they can read written instructions.
  (g) The patient and family's needs for information, support and education about the central venous line.
  (h) The patient's job and work environment, leisure and social activities.
  (i) The patient's home environment and facilities (e.g. the availability of a clean designated area for storage and preparation of equipment and drugs).

(2) The unit-based nurse plans and implements care in conjunction with the patient, family and other members of the multidisciplinary team.

  (a) The patient and family are provided with information and education related to:

  - the day-to-day management of the line (e.g. flushing the line)
  - the care of the exit and entry sites (e.g. daily shower)
  - principles of hygiene (e.g. handwashing)
  - what action to take if difficulties/problems arise
  - general symptoms/problems to observe for and report (e.g. cuff exposure, painful shoulder).

  (b) The nurse demonstrates care of the line to the patient and family, and supervises them in the initial stages of caring for the line themselves.
  (c) The nurse assesses both the competence and confidence of the patient and/or family in caring for the line.
  (d) The patient and family are offered support tailored to their individual and changing needs.
  (e) The patient and family are provided with written information related to the patient's treatment and the care of a central venous line.
  (f) The nurse assesses the exit and entry sites and the line daily, uses an aseptic technique when handling the line, assesses the patency of the line and on each admission checks the measurement from the exit site to the end of the line.
  (g) The nurse ensures that on discharge the patient has available a supply of all the correct equipment.

(3) The unit-based nurse monitors and evaluates the effectiveness of care as in (1) and the appropriateness of interventions to meet individual needs.

(4) The unit-based nurse will identify the need to refer the patient to other members of the multidisciplinary team, will act where necessary as co-ordinator of the multidisciplinary team and will communicate appropriate information.

NURSING

(5) The unit-based nurse facilitates continuity of care on discharge/transfer consulting with the clinical nurse specialist (outpatient chemotherapy) and the community liaison nurse where indicated and ensuring that the patient and/or family have a contact name or number for follow-up advice and support.

(6) The unit-based nurse documents accurately all aspects of professional practice.

5. OUTCOMES

(1) The patient and family feel that they were able to care safely and felt confident in the care of the central venous line, both in the hospital and on return home. They also feel that their needs for education and for emotional and practical support were met.

(2) The nurse considers that he or she had access to the resources as listed and was able to follow the described professional practice. The nurse also considers that, through the provision of education, information and support he or she was able to meet the needs of the patient and family enabling them to be competent and feel confident in the care of the central venous line. The nurse also considers that catheter patency was maintained and that there was prevention, early detection or minimization of complications.

(3) The documentation system will show evidence that resources were used and professional practice followed to ensure catheter patency, the prevention, early detection and minimization of complications and that the patient and/or family were competent and confident in the care of the central venous line. There will also be evidence that the patient and family's needs for education and for emotional and practical support were met.

REFERENCES AND FURTHER READING

Clarke, J. & Cox, E. (1988) Hepinarisation of Hickman catheters. *Nursing Times*, **84(15)**, (April 13), 51–3.

Johnstone, J. D. (1982) Infrequent infections associated with Hickman catheters. *Cancer Nursing*, **April**, 125–9.

Maki, D. G., Ringer, M. & Alvavadro, C. J. (1991) Prospective randomised trial of povidone-iodine, alcohol and chlorhexidine for the prevention of infection associated with central venous and arterival catheters. *The Lancet*, **338**, 339–42.

Milne, C. (1988) Hickman catheters. *Nursing Standard*, **3(8)**, (November 19).

Petrosino, B., Becker, H. & Christian, B. (1988) Infection rates in central venous catheter dressings. *Oncology Nursing Forum*, **15(6)**, 709–17.

Press, O. W., Ramsey, P. G., Larson, E. B., Fefor, A. & Hickman, R. O. (1984) Hickman catheter infections in patients with malignancies. *Medicine*, **63(4)**, 189–200.

CARING FOR CHILDREN AND THEIR FAMILIES ON ARRIVAL TO THE WARD

1. STANDARD STATEMENT

The nursing care of children and their families on arrival/admission to the paediatric unit, aims to provide a welcoming and friendly greeting to help alleviate anxiety and to establish good rapport as the basis of building an open and supportive relationship with nursing staff.

2. RATIONALE

Hospitalization can be a very difficult experience for children as they find themselves in an unfamiliar environment staffed by strangers. Rodin (1983) explains that several factors seem to have a major influence on a child's reaction to hospital. The first of these is separation of the child from his parents. Bowlby (1953) stated that a child should experience a warm, intimate and continuous relationship with the mother or mother substitute, and held that the young child who is immature in mind and body cannot cope with 'maternal' deprivation. Bowlby claims this can happen in hospital when 'maternal deprivation' can have far-reaching effects on the child's character development. Secondly, Olds (1978) considered the importance of humanizing the physical environment of the paediatric ward and stated that it is unlikely that children can disassociate medical procedures from uninviting and frightening circumstances which may surround some examinations and treatments. Comfortable child-orientated surroundings help to lower the child's anxiety (Olds, 1978) and a welcoming environment also helps in meeting the immediate needs of the parents. Furthermore the Court Report (1976) emphasized that the paediatric ward is the unit replacing home as far as the child in hospital is concerned, and advocated a child and family-centred philosophy of care.

The nurse plays a key role in developing a welcoming and friendly atmosphere and in assessing the immediate needs of both the child and their family.

3. RESOURCES

(1) The key worker (nurse) responsible for the child's admission will be a Registered Sick Children's Nurse or a second level nurse with paediatric training, with an oncology certificate/equivalent experience.

(2) The unit-based nurse will have a baseline knowledge of the following.

    (a) Paediatric malignancies and their treatment.
    (b) The psychological and social impact of the disease, its treatment and admission to hospital, on the child and family.
    (c) The impact of admission to hospital and the importance of first impressions to the child and family.
    (d) Family dynamics and functioning.
    (e) Child development.
    (f) The physical, emotional and behavioral signs of psychological distress (e.g. anxiety) in both children and adults.

(3) The unit-based nurse will have baseline skills in:

    (a) Communication – listening and observational skills in order to be receptive to both verbal and non-verbal cues and skills to establish good rapport with both the child and family.

(b) Teaching – to provide the child and family with appropriate information and to orientate them to the ward gradually.

(c) Practical techniques – for example, to provide immediate symptom control (where necessary).

(4) The unit-based nurse will have access to ongoing education and support. The clinical nurse specialist/unit manager will organize supervision, and unit-based teaching sessions, where necessary.

(5) The clinical nurse specialist (paediatrics) will have detailed knowledge and skills as listed in (1) and (2), and will be available to act as a resource or source of referral within the unit and throughout the hospital.

(6) Other members of the multidisciplinary team will be available to act as a resource or source of referral to the child, family and nurse including members of the child's medical team, registration staff/ward clerk and the play therapist.

(5) A range of equipment will be available, including:

(a) For the child (or siblings/friends where appropriate)

- suitable bedding
- a wide variety of toys, books and games
- television (in every bedroom and playroom)
- video cassette player and variety of videos

(b) For the parents

- use of folding bed
- access to kitchen equipment, including microwave, cooker, blender, kettles, fridge and freezer, and various utensils
- access to TV and video
- books, games and magazines.

(6) An environment suitable to the needs of the child (and siblings) will be available. It should be clean, uncluttered and decorated appropriately, for example with bright colours, pictures, mobiles etc. The environment must be safe for the individual child (e.g. locked cupboards, high door handles etc.) and should include the child's bed/cot space prepared before his or her arrival, availability of single room (where necessary) and access to a playroom.

(7) An environment suitable to the needs of the parents will be available. This should include space for one parent to sleep on the ward and access to a sitting room, a kitchen, laundry facilities and bathroom facilities.

4. PROFESSIONAL PRACTICE

(1) The unit-based nurse makes an initial assessment including the following.

(a) The child's name, age, diagnosis and where he or she is being admitted from (prior to their arrival, where possible).

(b) The child's general physical condition in order to identify symptoms requiring immediate treatment (e.g. pain, breathlessness).

(c) The immediate 'comfort' needs of the child and family (e.g. Are they tired? Are they hungry/thirsty?).

(d) The immediate psychological needs of the child and family (e.g. needs for privacy, information, time alone).

(e) The child's developmental stage.

(f) Signs of anxiety in both the child and family members.

(g) Family relationships and dynamics, including the sick child, parent(s) and sibling(s).

(2) The unit-based nurse plans and implements care in conjunction with other members of the multidisciplinary team.

(3) Prior to the child's arrival:

(a) All nursing staff and the ward clerk are made aware of the expected admission and basic details (name, age, etc.)

(b) A nurse is allocated to greet, admit and care for the child and family for that shift.

(c) An appropriate bed area, including any necessary equipment, is prepared.

(d) The allocated nurse will make any necessary preparation if diagnostic tests, treatment, etc. are planned for the day of admission.

(4) On arrival to the ward:

(a) The child and family are greeted by name – the nurse establishes how they wish to be addressed.

(b) The nurse introduces herself.

(c) Where necessary, the nurse liaises with medical staff to facilitate the prompt treatment of physical symptoms.

(d) The child is given the ward's introductory information booklet.

(e) The nurse explains the order of events for the child's first day in hospital to both the child and family.

(f) Depending on the individual child and family (e.g. their anxiety levels, the child's age, etc.) the nurse may show them to the prepared bed area, escort them to the playroom or show them around the ward.

(g) The nurse will introduce other staff and families as appropriate to individual needs.

(5) The unit-based nurse evaluates the effectiveness of interventions by reassessment as in (1).

(6) The nurse communicates appropriate information based on the initial assessment and evaluation to other relevant members of the multidisciplinary team.

(7) The unit-based nurse documents accurately all aspects of professional practice.

5. OUTCOMES

(1) The child and/or family report that they were greeted in a welcoming and friendly manner and that helped to establish a good rapport with the nursing staff. They also report that their immediate physical, informational and support needs were met.

(2) The nurse considers that he or she had access to resources as listed and was able to follow the described professional practice. The nurse also considers that he or she was able to greet the child and family in a welcoming and friendly manner and that this helped to alleviate their anxiety and establish good rapport with the nursing staff. They

NURSING

also report that the child and family's immediate physical, informational and support needs were met.

(3) The documentation system will show that resources were used and professional practice followed in order that the child and family were greeted in a welcoming and friendly manner and that their immediate physical, informational and support needs were met.

REFERENCES

Bowlby, J. (1953) *Child Care and the Growth of Love*. Penguin, Harmondsworth.
Court Report (1976) Committee on Child Health Services: Fit for the future. HMSO, London.
Olds, A. R. (1978) Humanising paediatric outpatient and hospital settings. In *Psychological Aspects of Paediatric Care*, (Ed. by E. Gellert), pp. 111–32. Grune & Stratton, New York.
Rodin, J. (1983) *Will this Hurt?* Royal College of Nursing, London.

CARE OF PATIENTS EXPERIENCING CHRONIC PAIN

NURSING

1. STANDARD STATEMENT

Patients who are experiencing chronic pain(s) will receive nursing care directed towards controlling or relieving this symptom to achieve optimum quality of life for each individual patient.

2. RATIONALE

Pain is the most common symptom in patients with advanced cancer (Twycross & Lack, 1983). Research evidence suggests that pain relief can be achieved for 85% of cancer patients who report pain as a symptom (WHO, 1986). Chronic pain is a complex subjective experience caused by complicated underlying mechanisms. A strong affective component – fear, anxiety or depression – may also be present and can have a profound isolating effect on patients and their ability to cope.

The principles of symptom management are to diagnose the mechanism of the pain problem, to individualize the treatment and to keep the treatment simple. During pain assessment, information is gathered from the patient which guides the planning and evaluation of nursing strategies for care. Pain is rarely static, therefore its assessment must be ongoing. Nursing interventions such as positioning, distraction and touch, in conjunction with pharmacological therapies, progressively aim to ensure that the patient is pain free at night, pain free at rest and pain free on movement. Nurses are in a key position to ensure that pain management is approached from a holistic perspective and meets individual patient needs.

Pain control is not just the responsibility of the nurse. Communication between health care colleagues and the utilization of the skills and knowledge of the multidisciplinary team are fundamental in offering successful symptom control. It is, however, the responsibility of the nurse to be aware of the range of supportive measures available and to refer to colleagues as appropriate.

3. RESOURCES

(1) The unit-based nurse will have a baseline knowledge of the following.

    (a) Assessing pain (taking into account physical, emotional and spiritual components).

    (b) The use of a pain assessment chart.

    (c) The use of pharmacological/non-pharmacological therapies available for the alleviation of pain (e.g. WHO, 1986, *The Royal Marsden Hospital Manual of Clinical Nursing Procedures* Chapter pp. 31, 349–54 & Chapter 38, pp. 435–41).

    (d) The appropriate use of prescribed variable doses of analgesia, including the titration of medication dosage against pain.

    (e) The chronic pains arising from malignant disease (as distinguished from acute pain).

    (f) The factors influencing pain – for example anxiety, isolation, insomnia (which lower pain threshold) and relaxation, diversional therapy, adequate sleep (which raise pain threshold).

    (g) The physical and psychological impact of chronic pain on the patient.

    (h) The impact of chronic pain on the patient's work, social and leisure activities.

    (i) Current research and trends in the management of chronic pain, and their implications for both the patient and family and related nursing care.

NURSING

(2) The unit-based nurse will have baseline skills in:

    (a) Communication – both verbal and written skills, for effective communication with the patient, family and other health professionals to assess and manage pain effectively.

    (b) Teaching – for effective individualized education of patient and family as to the causes of pain(s), therapies available and use of such therapies.

    (c) Practical techniques – for example in drug administration, setting up and using heat pads, distraction therapy, comfortable positioning etc.

(3) The unit-based nurse will have access to ongoing education and support. The clinical nurse specialist/unit manager will organize supervision, and unit-based teaching sessions, where necessary.

(4) The clinical nurse specialist/unit manager is expected to have detailed knowledge as listed in (1) and skills as in (2). Where the problem has specific management issues/difficulties, or has become persistent and intractable, a clinical nurse specialist/unit manager with specialist knowledge and skills may be identified to act as a consultant for advice and support.

(5) There will be a member of the patient's medical team available to discuss the symptom with the patient, the family and the nurse, who will be able to prescribe pharmacological therapy to ensure that an optimum level of symptom control is obtained.

(6) Other members of the multidisciplinary team will be available who may be a resource or source of referral to the patient, the family and nurse including the physiotherapist, occupational therapist, chaplain and social worker.

(7) There will be a range of pharmacological/non-pharmacological therapies and aids available.

(8) A range of appropriate written information booklets will be available to the patient and family.

(9) An environment suitable for the patient and family's needs and requirements should be made available wherever possible, and should include privacy, quiet etc.

(10) An environment suitable for the nurse's needs should be made available wherever possible (e.g. undisturbed time while preparing controlled drugs).

4. PROFESSIONAL PRACTICE

(1) The unit-based nurse makes an initial and ongoing assessment of the following.

    (a) The history of pain(s), including alleviation and exacerbation.

    (b) Pharmacological/non-pharmacological history including radiotherapy, surgery, etc.

    (c) The patient's own description of pain(s), using a pain assessment chart where appropriate.

    (d) Current presence, site and severity of pain(s).

    (e) Current factors influencing pain.

(2) Realistic treatment options are discussed and care is planned in conjunction with the patient, family and other members of the multidisciplinary team:

- Aiming for the patient to be pain free at night
- Aiming for the patient to be pain free at rest
- Aiming for the patient to be pain free on movement.

(3) The unit-based nurse plans and implements care in conjunction with the patient, family and other members of the multidisciplinary team.

    (a) Having identified factors which may be influencing the patient's pain, nursing interventions are implemented which are aimed at maximizing the patient's pain threshold, thereby relieving pain. These may include providing psychological support to relieve anxiety, promoting adequate rest and sleep, providing diversional activities, etc.

    (b) In collaboration with medical colleagues, the unit-based nurse ensures that an appropriate dose range of analgesia is prescribed (if necessary).

    (c) The unit-based nurse administers appropriate pharmacological therapies based on the nursing and medical assessments. According to his or her professional judgement, the nurse may vary the dose of analgesia given (within the prescribed range) depending on the patient's level of pain and activity.

    (d) The unit-based nurse teaches the patient and family how to use the pain assessment chart (if appropriate) and/or regularly updates the pain assessment chart (if used).

    (e) The unit-based nurse offers appropriate individualized information to the patient and family regarding treatment plans.

(4) The unit-based nurse monitors and evaluates the effectiveness of care as in (1) and the appropriateness of interventions to meet individual needs.

(5) The unit-based nurse will identify the need to refer the patient to other members of the multidisciplinary team, will act where necessary as a co-ordinator of the multi-disciplinary team and will communicate appropriate information.

(6) The unit-based nurse will facilitate continuity of care following discharge/transfer consulting with the community liaison nurse where indicated.

(7) The unit-based nurse documents accurately all aspects of professional practice.

---

5. OUTCOMES

(1) The patient and family report that the patient's pain was reduced/controlled. They also feel that their needs for education, and for practical and emotional support, were met.

(2) The nurse considers that he or she had access to the resources as listed and was able to follow the described professional practice. The nurse also reports that the patient's pain was reduced or controlled. The nurse also considers that the patient and family's needs for education and for practical and emotional support were met.

(3) The documentation system will show evidence that resources were used and professional practice followed to demonstrate that the patient's pain was reduced or controlled. There will be evidence that the patient and family's needs for education and for emotional and practical support were met.

REFERENCES

Twycross, R. G. & Lack, S. A. (1983) *Symptom Control in Advanced Cancer: Pain Relief.* Pitman, London.

World Health Organization (1986) *Cancer Pain Relief.* WHO, Geneva.

CARE OF PATIENTS EXPERIENCING CONSTIPATION

1. STANDARD STATEMENT

The nursing care of patients whose normal bowel pattern is or may become compromised resulting in constipation is directed towards the promotion of a realistic and acceptable elimination pattern for each individual patient.

2. RATIONALE

Constipation is an undue delay in faecal evacuation. It is the result of complex interactions of physical, social and psychological factors and treatment modalities which may include surgery, chemotherapy, inactivity, change in diet, inadequate fluid intake, depression, metabolic disorders (e.g. hypercalcaemia, hypokalaemia), neurological changes (e.g. spinal cord compression) and pharmacological effects (Portenoy, 1987). The patient may experience symptoms including nausea, headache, abdominal cramping or distention (Heitkemper & Bartol, 1986) and if unmanaged may lead to fecal impactation, severe discomfort and interference with daily living. Constipation is a common and distressing symptom in patients with cancer (Portenoy, 1987) and, for many, provokes great anxiety.

A key nursing role is the identification of patients at risk of, or experiencing constipation and in collaboration with the multidisciplinary team to offer appropriate treatment. Simple and therapeutic interventions should be instituted. Wherever possible, constipation should be anticipated and prevented through the use of prophylactic therapies. Patient awareness and education are crucial to maintain effective prevention and treatment (Catalano & Levy, 1985). Therefore, nursing care encompasses interventions which not only identify, treat or prevent constipation but which also enable the patient to adapt and cope.

3. RESOURCES

(1) The unit-based nurse will have a baseline knowledge of the following.

    (a) Factors causing constipation, including cancer and its treatment, the effects of various pharmacological therapies (e.g. opiods, antacids), metabolic disorders and psychological factors.

    (b) The physical and psychological effects of constipation (e.g. nausea, loss of appetite, low mood, lethargy, etc.).

    (c) The potential complications of constipation (e.g. bowel obstruction).

    (d) The non-pharmacological methods of preventing and/or relieving constipation (e.g. high fibre diet, exercise).

    (e) The pharmacological agents available for the treatment of constipation and their appropriate use.

    (f) Essential aspects of stoma management.

    (g) Current research and trends in the management of constipation, and their implications for both the patient and family and for related nursing care.

(2) The unit-based nurse will have baseline skills in:

    (a) Communication – for effective communication with the patient and family to ensure accurate assessment and management of the problem and treatment appropriate to the needs of the individual.

    (b) Teaching – for effective education of the patient and family regarding self-medication, methods of preventing constipation, and patterns of elimination.

NURSING

    (c) Practical techniques – in the administration of medications, in providing assistance with mobility, hygiene and special dietary requirements (to prevent constipation) and in essential aspects of stoma management.

(3) The unit-based nurse will have access to ongoing education and support. The clinical nurse specialist/unit manager will organize supervision, and unit-based teaching sessions, where necessary.

(4) The clinical nurse specialist/unit manager is expected to have detailed knowledge as listed in (1) and skills as in (2). Where the problem has specific management issues/difficulties or has become persistent and intractable a clinical nurse specialist/unit manager with specialist knowledge and skills may be identified to act as a consultant for advice and support.

(5) Other members of the multidisciplinary team will be available to act as a source of referral or resource to the patient, family and nurse including medical staff, dietitian, pharmacist, stomatherapist and appliance officer.

(6) There will be a range of equipment (e.g. commodes, gloves, bedpan washer) and treatments (e.g. effective pharmacological therapies, appropriate diet) for the prevention and treatment of constipation.

(7) Written information about diet and self-medication (including self-medication charts) will be available.

(8) An environment suitable to the patient's individual needs will be available (e.g. ensuring privacy, easy access to toilet and wash basin, etc.)

(9) An environment suitable to the needs of the nurse will be available (e.g. access to an appropriately equipped sluice).

---

4. PROFESSIONAL PRACTICE

(1) The unit-based nurse makes an initial and ongoing assessment of the following.

    (a) Any previous history of constipation and its alleviation/exacerbation.
    (b) The patient's usual bowel pattern.
    (c) Factors which may cause the patient to be constipated, including his or her disease and its treatment, any other drug therapy, physiological factors such as dehydration or hypercalcaemia and psychological factors such as depression.
    (d) The patient's previous and current dietary and fluid intake.
    (e) Whether the patient is currently constipated or at risk of constipation (including events leading up to constipation where appropriate).
    (f) The patient's mobility (e.g. whether he or she is able to walk to the toilet unaided/with help, etc.) and ability to exercise.
    (g) Physiological effects of constipation on the patient (e.g. nausea, loss of appetite, etc.)
    (h) The educational needs of the patient and family concerning the prevention and management of constipation.

(2) The unit-based nurse discusses care in conjunction with the patient, family and other relevant members of the multidisciplinary team:

- to prevent constipation (wherever possible)
- to promote a realistic and acceptable bowel pattern for the patient.

(3) The unit-based nurse plans and implements care in conjunction with the patient, family and other members of the multidisciplinary team.

   (a) Where constipation is likely to be a recurrent problem, the aim is to provide symptomatic relief and to help the patient and family cope with and adapt to the problem, for example by promoting an appropriate diet and fluid intake etc.
   (b) The unit-based nurse administers pharmacological and non-pharmacological therapies taking into account individual patient preference wherever possible.
   (c) The unit-based nurse provides prompt assistance for those patients needing help to the toilet, to use a commode or bedpan or assistance with personal hygiene, taking into account the patients' individual needs for privacy and dignity.

(4) The unit-based nurse monitors and evaluates the effectiveness of care as in (1) and the appropriateness of interventions to meet individual needs.

(5) The unit-based nurse will identify the need to refer the patient to other members of the multidisciplinary team where appropriate, will act where necessary as a co-ordinator of the multidisciplinary team and communicate appropriate information.

(6) The unit-based nurse will facilitate continuity of care following discharge/transfer, consulting with the community liaison nurse where indicated.

(7) The unit-based nurse documents accurately all aspects of professional practice.

5. OUTCOMES

(1) The patient and family report that a realistic and acceptable elimination pattern was achieved in accordance with the patient's individual needs. They also report that their needs for education and for practical and emotional support were met.

(2) The nurse reports that he or she had access to the resources as listed and was able to follow the described professional practice. The nurse also considers that an acceptable elimination pattern was achieved for the patient to meet his or her individual needs and that the patient and family's needs for education and for practical and emotional support were met.

(3) The documentation system will show evidence that resources were used and professional practice followed to promote a realistic and acceptable elimination pattern for the patient meeting his or her individual needs. There will also be evidence that the patient and family's needs for education and for practical and emotional support were met.

REFERENCES

Catalano, R. B. & Levy, M. H. (1985) Control of common physical symptoms other than pain in the patient with terminal disease. *Seminars in Oncology*, **12(4)**, 411–30.
Heitkemper, P. & Bartol, K. (1986) Gastrointestinal problems. In *Nursing Management for the Elderly*, 2nd edn (Ed. by D. Carnevali & M. Patrick), J.B. Lippincott, Philadelphia.
Portenoy, R. K. (1987) Constipation in the cancer patient. *Medical Clinics of North America*, **71(2)**, 303–11.

CARE OF PATIENTS WITH CULTURALLY SPECIFIC HEALTH NEEDS

1. STANDARD STATEMENT

The nursing care of patients and families with culturally specific health needs is directed towards facilitating communication, demonstrating awareness of and respect for their beliefs and practices and wherever possible accommodating these practices.

2. RATIONALE

When the National Health Service was established in 1948 it was designed to care for the needs of the indigenous population. Today health service provision and staff training programmes are still geared to this way of life with the present design of the services geared almost exclusively to the needs, values and expectations of the indigenous population (London Association of Community Councils, 1985, National Association of Health Authorities, 1988). Over the last 30 years, however, the composition of the population in many areas has changed significantly and so have health needs. Britain today is a multiracial, multicultural and multi-religious society. People from different ethnic origins continue to maintain their customs, cultural heritage and religious beliefs.

There has been a growing feeling among professionals and community organizers that the policies and structures of the NHS have helped to prevent an adequate response to the health needs of the ethnic minority populations (Mares et al., 1985). The Commission for Racial Equality (1989) considers that the proposals of the White Paper on the review of the NHS do little to improve or amend the provision of services to make them more appropriate and adequate to the needs of ethnic minority groups. For example, funding changes recommended by the White Paper are based on population number and are weighted for health, age, morbidity and the relative costs of providing care to that population. The suggested changes do not incorporate inclusion of cultural considerations (Commission for Racial Equality, 1989).

In recent years there has been increasing focus on the health of the British black and ethnic minority communities (Baxter, 1989). It is well established that this sector of the population has a worse health experience than the majority white population (Torkington, 1983, Marmot et al., 1984, Fenton, 1985). The increase in the ethnic diversity of countries has put demands on the health care system to provide care which is culturally acceptable as well as effective and economical (Anderson, 1990). The NHS Act (1977) states that:

'it is every Health Authority's duty ... to arrange as with respects their area ... to provide personal medical services for all persons in the area who wish to take advantage of the arrangements'.

There is evidence that people from black and ethnic minority groups have higher than average mortality rates from common medical disorders (Marmot et al., 1981, OPCS, 1985, Nikolaides et al. 1985, Mather & Keen, 1985). The experience of cancer in these communities has received little attention; information and research are scant. Various studies in the United States have highlighted that the pattern of malignancy after one or two generations of migration takes on the same pattern as the majority population. Similar studies have also confirmed that black people, for example, are consistently diagnosed at a later clinical stage (McWorther & Mayer, 1987) and as a consequence tend to have poorer experiences and survival rates (Axtell & Myers, 1978, Nemeto et al., 1980, Bassett & Kreiger, 1986). The literature tends to concentrate on mainly diagnosis and clinical aspects of care and not on secondary or tertiary aspects of care such as access to hospices and support of carers.

The cultural variations in patient population have also increased the complexity of caring, and demand an understanding that usually goes beyond the traditional preparation of nurses (Anderson, 1987). When a person has cancer, complex factors influence how this experience is perceived and related to – cultural aspects are one of these factors. Research has highlighted the need for nurses to be more attentive to the cultural and social context of health care (Anderson & Chung, 1982, Anderson et al. 1989). Sampson (1982), for example, highlights what she refers to as the neglected ethic:

> 'The nurse in providing care promotes an environment in which the values, customs and spiritual beliefs of the individual are respected'.
>
> (ICN Code of Nursing Ethics)

She believes that nurses do not deliberately neglect the customs or beliefs of patients but simply lack the necessary knowledge and skills.

Although attentiveness to one's values is critical in all relationships, it takes on highlighted importance when nurse and patient are from different cultural groups, where cultural beliefs and values are more likely to differ. For nurses to be able to assess a patient's needs accurately and implement appropriate care, there is need to acknowledge cultural and religious differences (Barclay, 1990). This belief is supported by Anderson (1987) who considers that the key to providing culturally sensitive care is firstly that the nurse is aware of both his/her own culture, values and beliefs and recognize that these may come in the way of caring. Nurses are influenced by their own professional culture as well as by their own personal values.

Through the process of interview, nurses should be able to elicit cultural as well as social data. Thorough assessment can avoid stereotyping. Culture is not static and in practice very few people respond to the total stereotype (Sampson, 1982). There are variations between social groups within one culture illustrating a diversity of attitudes, behaviour and expectations. Assessment needs to incorporate patients' perceptions of health and illness including the interpretation of their current illness and any symbolic meanings related to that, and their notions about treatment, the use of traditional remedies and practitioners, the patient and family's perceptions of nurses and hospitals, and their perceptions of care in hospital and the role of the family (Anderson, 1987). Nurses also need to consider the range of aspects of care that are influenced by cultural factors such as diet, bereavement, clothing, drugs and alcohol. Nurses, therefore, play a major role in both the assessment of cultural needs and ensuring culturally sensitive care is provided for all patients.

---

3. RESOURCES

(1) The unit-based nurse will have a baseline knowledge/awareness of the following.

   (a) The various religious/cultural backgrounds of patients admitted to the unit.
   (b) How and where to obtain information concerning specific religious and cultural beliefs and practices.
   (c) Certain political and religious difficulties/differences and their implications for the patient and nursing care (e.g. when allocating patients to a shared room).
   (d) The resources available to patients and families who have difficulty speaking/ understanding English (e.g. Red Cross language cards, cultural and religious organizations, translators, embassies etc.)
   (e) The resources available to patients and families with specific needs related to their cultural/religious background (e.g. spiritual needs, dietary requirements, etc.)
   (f) Differences in health beliefs, illness behaviour and perception between cultures – for example, aiming for self-care may not always be practical or appropriate.
   (g) The various cultural/religious practices associated with death, dying and bereavement.

(h) The implications of cultural and/or religious beliefs and practices for activities of daily living (e.g. specific beliefs concerning privacy and dignity, hygiene practices etc.) and for treatment (e.g. shaving, use of prostheses etc.).

(i) The need to respect and accommodate cultural/religious needs related to social behaviour (e.g. eating habits) and the social organization of the family/group (e.g. care-giving roles, whom to give information etc.).

(j) The importance of dietary requirements/restrictions due to religious practices, and how these may be met during hospitalization.

(k) The potential psychological, social and financial impact of cancer, its treatment and side-effects on the individual and family (e.g. altered body image, role change, etc.).

(l) The potential psychological impact of being separated from one's home culture or country and/or family group members.

(2) The unit-based nurse will have baseline skills in:

(a) Communication – the use of non-verbal and listening skills (including using charts, pictures, simple sign language etc.), and recognition of non-verbal cues. The nurse should be aware that non-verbal signs may have different meanings within different cultures.

(b) Teaching – to offer information to the patient and/or family about the disease and its treatment (where possible and appropriate).

(c) Practical techniques – and be able to demonstrate practical skills to the patient and/or family.

(3) The unit-based nurse will have access to ongoing education and support. The clinical nurse specialist/unit manager will organize supervision, and unit-based teaching sessions, where necessary.

(4) The clinical nurse specialist/unit manager is expected to have detailed knowledge as listed in (1) and skills as in (2). Where the problem has specific management issues/difficulties a clinical nurse specialist/unit manager with specialist knowledge and skills may be identified to act as a consultant for advice and support.

(5) Other members of the multidisciplinary team will be available to act as a source of referral or resource to the patient, family and nurse including dietitians, catering managers, physiotherapists, chaplains and speech therapists.

(6) Written information will be available to the patient and family including general information on the hospital, information on proposed treatments and their implications, information about organizations outside the hospital etc. There will also be a range of such information in a variety of languages for those patients and families who either cannot, or have difficulty in, understanding written English.

(7) Written information will be available to the nurse including access to information about various religions and cultures and their related practices, a directory of interpreters, a directory of embassy telephone numbers and contact names, and information about the Community Relations Council, etc.

(8) An environment suitable to the needs of the patient (and family) will be available wherever possible (e.g. access to privacy in order to pray, access to running water in order to meet both hygiene and religious requirements).

(9) An environment to meet the needs/requirements of the nurse will be available (e.g. access to single room where possible for information giving).

4. PROFESSIONAL PRACTICE

(1) The unit-based nurse makes an initial and ongoing assessment of the following:

(a) The patient's cultural and religious background.

(b) The patient and family's understanding of both written and spoken English, and ability to communicate through the spoken word.

(c) The need to accommodate any practices associated with the patient and/or family's cultural or religious background.

(d) The psychological impact for the patient and family of being separated from their own culture/country.

(e) The dietary requirements of the patient.

(f) The level of family support and the family's needs, willingness and ability to participate in care.

(g) The implications of both the disease and the proposed treatment on the patient's customs, cultural and religious practices.

(2) The unit-based nurse plans and implements care in conjunction with the patient, family and other members of the multidisciplinary team.

(a) The nurse ensures that the dietary requirements of the patient are addressed, liaising with the dietitian and catering department as necessary.

(b) The nurse ensures that wherever possible the cultural/religious practices of the patient are accommodated and religious/cultural beliefs respected (e.g. allowing patients to wear headcoverings or wristbands to theatre, planning the administration of chemotherapy so as not to coincide with times of prayer, etc.)

(c) The family are encouraged to be involved in care wherever possible. Where appropriate the nurse liaises with the 'spokesperson' of the family.

(d) The nurse ensures wherever possible that the language needs of the patient are met, and arranges an interpreter as necessary.

(e) Where possible patients are introduced to other patients with similar cultural backgrounds or needs if this is acceptable to both groups.

(3) The unit-based nurse monitors and evaluates the effectiveness of care as in (1) and the appropriateness of interventions to meet individual needs.

(4) The unit-based nurse will identify the need to refer the patient to other members of the multidisciplinary team, will act where necessary as co-ordinator of the multidisciplinary team and will communicate appropriate information to other professionals/departments about patients' cultural needs.

(5) The unit-based nurse will facilitate continuity of care on discharge/transfer, consulting with the family, embassies and the community liaison nurse where indicated. The patient and/or family are given a contact name or number for follow-up advice and support.

(6) The unit-based nurse documents accurately all aspects of professional practice.

5. OUTCOMES

(1) The patient and family report that communication was facilitated, awareness and respect demonstrated for their cultural/religious beliefs and practices, and that these

NURSING

practices were accommodated wherever possible. They will also feel that their needs for education and for emotional and practical support were met.

(2) The nurse considers that he or she had access to the resources as listed and was able to follow the described professional practice. The nurse also considers that communication was facilitated, awareness and respect demonstrated for the patient's cultural/religious beliefs and practices, and that these practices where accommodated wherever possible.

(3) The documentation system will show evidence that resources were used and professional practice followed to facilitate communication, demonstrate awareness and respect for cultural/religious beliefs and practices, and to accommodate these practices wherever possible. There will also be evidence that the patient and family's needs for education and for emotional and practical support were met.

REFERENCES

Anderson, J. & Chung, J. (1982) Culture and illness: parents' perceptions of their child's long term illness. *Nursing Papers*, **14** (winter), 40–52.

Anderson, J. M. (1987) The cultural context of caring. *Canadian Critical Care Nursing Journal*, **4** (December), 7–13.

Anderson, J. M. *et al.* (1989) Ideology in the clinical context: chronic illness, ethnicity and the discourse on normalization. *Journal of Social Medicine*, **11**, 253–78.

Anderson, J. M. (1990) Health Care Across Cultures. *Nursing Outlook*, **38(3)**, 136–9.

Axtell, L. M. & Myers, M. H. (1978) Contrasts in black and white cancer patients 1960–73. *JNCI*, **60**, 1209–1215.

Barclay, J. (1990) Transcultural nursing. Appendix 3 in *Ballière's Nurses Dictionary*, 21st edn (Ed. by B. F. Weller & R. J. Wells), pp. 518–24.

Bassett, M. T. & Kreiger, N. (1986) Social class and black and white differences in breast cancer survival. *American Journal of Public Health*, **76**, 1400–3.

Baxter, C. (1989) *Cancer Support and Ethnic Minority and Migrant Work Communities*. A summary of a research report commissioned by CancerLink.

Commission for Racial Equality (1989) *In Response to the Government's White Paper on the Review of the National Health Service*. CRE, London: p. 11.

Fenton, C. S. (1985) *Race, Wealth and Welfare – Afro-Caribbean and South Asian People in South Bristol*. Department of Sociology, University of Bristol.

International Council of Nurses. *Code of Nursing Ethics*. ICN, Geneva.

London Association for Community Relations Councils (1985) In *A Critical Condition*. LACRC, London.

Mares, P., Henley, A. & Baxter, C. (1985) *Health Care in Multiracial Britain*. Health Education Council/National Extension College Trust Ltd, Cambridge.

Marmot, M.G. *et al.* (1981) Cardiovascular mortality among immigrants to England and Wales. *Postgraduate Medical Journal*, December.

Marmot, M., Adelstein, A. & Bulusen, L. (1984) *Immigrant Mortality in England and Wales 1970–1978*, HMSO, London.

Mather, H. & Keen, H. (1985) The Southall Diabetics Survey: prevalence of known diabetes in Asians and Europeans. *British Medical Journal*, **291**, 19.

McWorther, W. P. & Mayer, W. J. (1987) Black and white differences in type of initial breast cancer treatment and implications for survival. *American Journal of Public Health*, **77(12)**.

National Association of Health Authorities (1988) *Action Not Words*. NAHA, London.

Nemeto, T., Vana, J., Bedivani, R. N. *et al.* (1980) Management and survival of female breast cancer: results of a national survey by the American College of Surgeons. *Cancer* **45**, 2917–24.

Nikolaides, K. *et al.* (1981) West Indian Diabetic Population of a Large Inner City Diabetic Clinic, *British Medical Journal*, November 21.

OPCS (1985) Infant and Perinatal Mortality 1983: *Birthweight*, DH 385/1 February.

Sampson, C. (1982) *The Neglected Ethic: Religious and Cultural Factors in the Care of Patients*. McGraw-Hill, London.

Torkington, W. P. K. (1983) *The Racial Politics of Health – A Liverpool Profile*. Merseyside Area Profile Group, Department of Epidemiology, University of Liverpool.

NURSING

CARE OF DYING PATIENTS AND THEIR FAMILIES

1. STANDARD STATEMENT

The nursing care of patients who are dying is directed towards maintaining patient dignity, respecting individuality, promoting physical comfort, and allowing patients and families choice, control and involvement in care wherever possible. Patients and families will be offered support and information to enable them to meet their physical, emotional, spiritual and social needs.

2. RATIONALE

Death remains one of the few certainties in life today. While death is a biological event, the experiences of dying are shaped by psychological, cultural and spiritual factors as well as physical ones (Neuberger, 1987). Each dying patient is unique and there is no ultimate guide for health care professionals (Brown, 1988). 'Even when dying a person can still have a sense of purpose and self esteem. The mode of dying will be as individual as the person himself' (Lamerton, 1973). Individuals and their families may respond to dying in a variety of ways. Some responses can be anticipated (Kubler Ross, 1970, James, 1989), while others cannot. Brown (1988) has summarized the needs of the dying patient as (1) the need to receive support based on an understanding of his/her task of adjusting to his/her dying; (2) the need to have relief from distressing physical symptoms; and (3) the need to know his/her family are supported and will continue to be so after the death.

Each patient has to do his own dying – we cannot do it for him (Stedeford, 1987). Nurses, however, can be instrumental in meeting patients' needs. Integral to care is the recognition of the subtle emotional, psychological and spiritual transitions that the patient needs to make in order to move through the dying process and along the dying continuum. Through detailed and perceptive assessment nurses can ease transition by being available to facilitate the process. Nurses play a key role offering individualized information and support, ensuring effective symptom control and promoting patient comfort. They are crucial members of the multidisciplinary team.

3. RESOURCES

(1) The unit-based nurse will have a baseline knowledge of the following.

   (a) Symptom control and the promotion of physical comfort.
   (b) The legal and ethical issues surrounding death and dying (e.g. signing of wills, death certification, the process and purpose of post mortem examination, the ethical controversies surrounding euthanasia, etc.)
   (c) Last offices according to the *Royal Marsden Hospital Manual of Clinical Nursing Procedures* (Chapter 23, pp. 280–85).
   (d) The cultural and religious influences on death and dying and the sources of advice and guidance prior to and in the event of death.
   (e) Patients' and families' fears concerning and their psychological reactions to death and dying.
   (f) Loss and bereavement, normal and abnormal grief reactions.
   (g) The role of other members of the multidisciplinary team in the management of death and dying.
   (h) Attitudes to death and dying and their influence on patient care.
   (i) Local and national services and resources available to support the dying individual and his or her family, in addition to services and resources available to the family following bereavement.

(2) The unit-based nurse will have baseline skills in:

(a) Communication – listening skills and observational skills, and skills in clarification to ensure that patients' needs are understood.
(b) Teaching – especially offering explanation and providing individualized information.
(c) Practical techniques – to promote physical comfort and involve families in care where appropriate.

(3) The unit-based nurse will have access to ongoing education and support. The clinical nurse specialist/unit manager will organize supervision, and unit-based teaching sessions, where necessary.

(4) The clinical nurse specialist/unit manager (continuing care) will have detailed knowledge as listed in (1) and skills as in (2). She or he will provide expert nursing care to patients who have intractable or persistant symptoms, are having difficulties coping with changes imposed by cancer, or whose families are in need of additional support. The clinical nurse specialist/unit manager will supervise the ward staff and act as a resource, educator and role model related to issues surrounding the dying process.

(5) Other members of the multidisciplinary team will be available to act as a resource or source of referral to the patient, family and nurse including chaplains, social workers, medical staff and the community liaison nurses.

(6) There will be a range of equipment and an environment to meet the needs of the patient, nurse and family.

4. PROFESSIONAL PRACTICE

(1) The unit-based nurse makes an initial and ongoing assessment of:

(a) The patient and family's understanding, feelings and perceptions of their disease status and prognosis, and their needs for information and support.
(b) The patient and family's cultural needs.
(c) The patient and family's spiritual needs.
(d) The patient and family's social needs.
(e) The patient and family's religious needs.
(f) The patient and family's physical needs.
(g) The family's willingness, ability and need to participate in the care of the patient and the appropriateness of such involvement.
(h) Whether the home or hospital environment is the most suitable for the patient to die in and the wishes of both the patient and family regarding this.

(2) The unit-based nurse plans and implements care in conjunction with the patient, family and other members of the multidisciplinary team.

(a) The nurse ensures that patient comfort is promoted and wherever possible symptom control achieved according to the patient's individual preferences.
(b) The nurse takes time to be with both the patient and the family.
(c) The nurse ensures that the patient and family's needs for privacy are respected.
(d) The nurse offers the patient and family information and support tailored to their individual and changing needs.
(e) The nurse teaches the patient skills related to self-care in order to maximize the patient's quality of life wherever possible.

(f) The nurse teaches, encourages and supports the family in their involvement in the care of the patient.

(g) The nurse ensures wherever possible that the patient and family have an appropriate level of information with which to make informed choices about their care.

(h) The nurse represents the patient's views either when the patient requests this or when the patient is no longer able to make decisions for him/herself.

(3) The nurse co-ordinates such interventions with other members of the multidisciplinary team to ensure that an optimum level of care is attained and maintained.

(4) The unit-based nurse monitors and evaluates the effectiveness of care as in (1) and the appropriateness of interventions to meet individual needs.

(5) The unit-based nurse will identify the need to refer the patient to other members of the multidisciplinary team, will act where necessary as co-ordinator of the multidisciplinary team, and will communicate appropriate information.

(6) The unit-based nurse will facilitate continuity of care on discharge/transfer, consulting with the community liaison nurses and the primary health care team where indicated, and ensuring that the patient and/or family have a contact name or number for advice and support.

(7) The unit-based nurse documents accurately all aspects of professional practice.

5. OUTCOMES

(1) The patient and/or family report that the patient's dignity was maintained and individuality respected and that the patient's physical comfort was promoted. They also feel that their needs for education and for emotional and practical support were met, and that wherever possible they were involved in care according to their individual wishes.

(2) The nurse considers that he or she had access to the resources as listed and was able to follow the described professional practice. The nurse also considers that the patient's dignity was maintained and individuality respected and that the patient's physical comfort was promoted. The nurse also considers that the patient and family's needs for education and for emotional and practical support were met, and that wherever possible they were involved in care according to their individual wishes.

(3) The documentation system will show evidence that resources were used and professional practice followed to maintain patient dignity, respect individuality, promote patient comfort, and allow choice, control and involvement in care wherever possible. There will also be evidence that the patient and family's needs for education and for emotional and practical support were met.

REFERENCES

Brown, J. (1988) Care of the dying. In *Nursing the Patient with Cancer*, (Ed. by V. Tschudin), pp. 409–36. Prentice Hall, Hemel Hempstead.

James, N. (1989) Emotional labour: skill and work in the social regulation of feelings. *Sociological Review*, **37(1)**, 15–42.

Lamerton, R. (1973) *Care of the Dying*. Penguin, Harmondsworth.

Kubler-Ross, E. (1970) *On Death and Dying*. Tavistock, London.

Marks, M. (1988) Death, dying, bereavement and loss. In *Oncology for Nurses and Health Care Professionals*, 2nd edn, Vol. 2, *Care and Support* (Ed. by R. Tiffany & P. Webb).

Neuberger, J. (1987) *Caring for Dying People of Different Faiths*. Lisa Sainsbury Foundation, Austen Cornish, Croydon.

Stedeford, A. (1987) Hospice: a safe place to suffer. *Palliative Medicine*, **1**, 73–4.

NURSING

CARE OF PATIENTS EXPERIENCING DYSPNOEA

1. STANDARD STATEMENT

Patients who are experiencing dyspnoea will receive nursing care directed towards the relief of distress and the promotion of comfort.

2. RATIONALE

Dyspnoea is the subjective feeling of not being able to breathe (Carrieri, 1986). It results when there is either increased ventilatory demand or decreased ventilatory capacity. In cancer patients both these factors may be present simultaneously, for example in a patient with fever (increased demand) and pleural effusion (decreased capacity) (Hoy, 1987).

Dyspnoea is a common symptom experienced by patients with advanced cancer. The statistics of two hospices, for example, show that half of all patients were admitted for dyspnoea. Another article reported that 22% of patients with advanced cancer utilized morphine for the primary relief of dyspnoea rather than the relief of pain (Hanks & Hoskins, 1988). Dyspnoea as a cause of suffering has been ranked with unrelieved pain yet is considered more difficult to palliate (Heyse-Moore, 1984). These three factors — high incidence, high degree of suffering and difficulty in palliation — make dyspnoea an important area for nursing care.

Such care focusses on facilitation of treatment of underlying causes through collaboration with the medical team; minimization of the symptom of dyspnoea through such approaches as massage, relaxation and distraction, and enabling the adaptation of patients and families so that lifestyle and priorities may be maintained. In order to achieve this, a multidisciplinary approach is essential to offer patients and families all that is available so that they may choose therapies that best suit their lifestyle, and promote quality of life as they define it.

3. RESOURCES

(1) The unit-based nurse will have a baseline knowledge of the following.

- (a) Disease processes causing dyspnoea.
- (b) Factors influencing dyspnoea (e.g. anxiety).
- (c) Pharmacological and non-pharmacological interventions.
- (d) The physical and psychological implications of dyspnoea for the patient and family.
- (e) The impact of dyspnoea on the patient's work, social and leisure activities.
- (f) Current research and trends in the management of dyspnoea and their implications for both the patient and family and for related nursing care.

(2) The unit-based nurse will have baseline skills in:

- (a) Communication — for effective communication with the patient and family to ensure accurate assessment of the problem and to relieve anxiety and distress (including distress of other members of staff).
- (b) Teaching — for effective education of the patient and family regarding comfortable positioning in bed or in a chair, to recognize activities or situations which may exacerbate breathlessness and the teaching of skills to manage the symptom.
- (c) Practical techniques — for example, in the administration of pharmacological and non-pharmacological therapies and providing assistance with positioning and mobility.

(3) The unit-based nurse will have access to ongoing education and support. The clinical nurse specialist/unit manager will organize supervision, and unit-based teaching sessions, where necessary.

(4) The clinical nurse specialist/unit manager is expected to have detailed knowledge as listed in (1) and skills as in (2). Where the problem has specific management issues/difficulties or has become persistent and intractable a clinical nurse specialist/unit manager with specialist knowledge and skills may be identified to act as a consultant for advice and support.

(5) Other members of the multidisciplinary team will be available to act as a source of referral or resource to the patient, family and nurse including medical staff, physiotherapists, occupational therapists and the therapeutic massage specialist.

(6) There will be a range of equipment and treatments for the relief of dyspnoea (e.g. oxygen and a variety of equipment for their administration, comfortable chairs, fans etc.)

(7) An environment suitable to the patient's individual needs will be available (e.g. a calm and quiet atmosphere).

4. PROFESSIONAL PRACTICE

(1) The unit-based nurse makes an initial and ongoing assessment of the following.

  (a) Previous history of dyspnoea and its alleviation/exacerbation.
  (b) Current presence of dyspnoea and systemic effects.
  (c) Factors which may cause the patient to be breathless, including disease status and associated systemic effects.
  (d) Current factors alleviating/exacerbating the symptom.
  (e) The patient's response to current pharmacological and non-pharmacological interventions.
  (f) The patient's mobility and optimum positioning for symptom relief.
  (g) The psychological effects of the symptom on the patient and family, and their needs for support.
  (h) The socioeconomic and practical factors likely to influence the patient's discharge home (e.g. the presence of stairs, the availability of family support).
  (i) The educational needs of the patient and family concerning the promotion of comfort and relief of distress.

(2) The unit-based nurse plans care in conjunction with the patient, family and other members of the multidisciplinary team:

  • to achieve optimal comfort
  • to maximize the reduction of dyspnoea and to relieve distress.

(3) Where dyspnoea is likely to be a recurrent or long term problem, the aim is to implement care that will provide symptomatic relief and to help the patient and family cope with and adapt to the problem.

  (a) The nurse identifies and alleviates (wherever possible) external factors exacerbating dyspnoea, e.g. noise, heat, claustrophobic situations, etc.
  (b) The nurse assists with patient positioning using aids where appropriate.
  (c) The nurse administers pharmacological therapies taking into account individual

NURSING

preferences where possible and liaising with the unit medical staff to ensure optimum symptom control.

(d) The nurse offers to teach both the patient and his or her family the use of breathing and relaxation exercises in relieving dyspnoea.

(e) The nurse offers support and reassurance to both the patient and family, for example by remaining with the patient at times of respiratory distress.

(f) The nurse provides prompt assistance with activities of daily living and advises the patient and family on reducing exertion while promoting maximum independence.

(10) The unit-based nurse monitors and evaluates the effectiveness of care as in (1) and the efficacy of interventions to meet individual needs.

(11) The unit-based nurse will identify the need to refer the patient to other members of the multidisciplinary team where appropriate, will act where necessary as co-ordinator of the multidisciplinary team and will communicate appropriate information.

(12) The unit-based nurse will facilitate continuity of care following discharge/transfer consulting with the community liaison nurse where indicated and ensuring that the patient and/or family have a contact name and number for follow-up advice and information.

(13) The unit-based nurse documents accurately all aspects of professional practice.

5. OUTCOMES

(1) The patient and family report that comfort was promoted and distress relieved in accordance with the patient's individual needs. They also consider that their needs for education and for practical and emotional support were met.

(2) The nurse reports that he or she had access to the resources as listed and was able to follow the described professional practice. The nurse also considers that comfort was promoted and distress relieved for the patient in order to meet her or his individual needs, and that the patient and family's need for education and for practical and emotional support were met.

(3) The documentation system will show evidence that resources were used and professional practice followed to promote patient comfort and relieve distress. There will be evidence that the patient and family's needs for education and for practical and emotional support were met.

REFERENCES

Carrieri, V. (1986) Dyspnoea. In *Pathophysiological Phenomena in Nursing*. (Ed. by V. Carrieri, A. Lindsey & C. West), pp. 191–218. W.B. Saunders, Philadelphia.

Hanks, G. & Hoskins, P. J. (1988) The management of symptoms in advanced cancer. Experience in a hospital-based continuing care unit. *Journal of the Royal Society of Medicine*, **81**, 341–4.

Heyse-Moore, L. (1984) Dyspnoea. In *The Management of Terminal Malignant Disease*, (Ed. by C. Saunders), pp. 113–19. Edward Arnold, London.

Hoy, A. M. (1987) Dyspnoea. *Baillière's Clinical Oncology*, Monograph **1(2)**.

CARE OF THE FAMILY OF CRITICALLY ILL PATIENTS

NURSING

1. STANDARD STATEMENT

The nursing care of the family of the critically ill patient is directed towards providing an open and supportive atmosphere or environment in which the family feels comfortable and able to be themselves. An integral part of nursing care is ensuring that the family, who are regarded as a holistic unit, are involved in and informed about both patient care and the decision making process to a degree that they determine.

2. RATIONALE

When a loved one becomes critically ill the family (including relatives, friends and significant others) may be thrown into a crisis situation (Daley, 1984). The normal family routine and relationships may be thrown into disarray and, initially, family members may undergo a period of disbelief, shock and may experience a sense of unreality (Stillwell, 1984, Coulter, 1988). In time physical, psychological and social reactions occur in response to the stress the family members undergo. These reactions may include an increase or decrease in crying, drinking, eating, sleeping and exercising. Individuals can also experience physical symptoms such as palpitations, backache, muscle tightness, constipation, migraine as well as somatic problems (Green, 1982). Within the family itself there can be withdrawal or the family can be drawn closer together; they may argue less or more and frequently feel isolated, helpless and hopeless (Brawlin *et al.*, 1982).

The family are also faced with very practical problems. Financial concerns are likely to arise, particularly if the critically ill person is the primary earner. There may also be difficulties with transport and arrangements for childcare. A spouse and children may undergo deprivation from their primary social contact, role changes and a period of mourning during the critical phase (Breu & Dracup, 1978).

The various essential needs of the family of a critically ill patient have been identified. These include the need for information given honestly and openly in terms understandable by the family (Molter & Captain, 1979) and, as Coulter (1988) suggests, this should be provided by the medical and nursing staff in immediate attendance of the patient. The need to be nearby or with the patient can be facilitated by open visiting and access to relatives' accommodation in the vicinity of the unit. The family also require relief from anxiety (Daley, 1984), to know the expected outcome from treatment and to have equipment explained. Religious and spiritual needs and the need for social support from friends and multidisciplinary team members must also be addressed wherever appropriate. Nurses play a key role in meeting these needs through the provision of information, education and support, and their invaluable role as co-ordinator of the multidisciplinary team.

3. RESOURCES

(1) The unit-based nurse will have a baseline knowledge of the following:

    (a) Family dynamics and functioning.
    (b) The physical, psychological and social implications of critical illness for the family.
    (c) The needs of the family of the critically ill patient.
    (d) The support systems and resources, both informal and formal, available to the family within the hospital and in the community.
    (e) The disease processes, treatments and equipment.

(2) The unit-based nurse will have baseline skills in:

(a) Communication – to provide accurate and effective information and to liaise with other members of the multidisciplinary team. The ability to listen to the family and to convey an individualized and empathetic attitude/approach is important too.

(b) Teaching – to teach the family patient care where appropriate.

(c) Practical techniques – to be responsive to the patient's needs whilst appearing confident and competent to the family.

(3) The unit-based nurse will have access to ongoing education and support. The clinical nurse specialist/unit manager will organize supervision, and unit-based teaching sessions, where necessary.

(4) The clinical nurse specialist/unit manager (HDU) will have detailed knowledge as listed in (1) and skills as in (2). She or he provides expert nursing care to family members during periods of acute crisis, supervises the ward staff and maintains a professional environment which supports the delivery of holistic and family centred care.

(5) Other members of the multidisciplinary team will be available to act as a resource or source of referral to the family and nurse including the medical staff, social workers, psychological support team, chaplains and translators.

(6) There will be a range of equipment available to the family including comfortable chairs, television, radio and equipment for making drinks and snacks.

(7) The nurse will have access to current written information and research including the nursing assessment form, a reference list of support groups and resources available to the family, information booklets and general textbooks related to oncology and critical care.

(8) Written information will be available to the patient and family including information about the high dependency unit, a range of booklets from *The Royal Marsden Hospital Patient Information Series* and information related to support groups and bereavement services.

(9) An environment suitable to the family's individual needs will be available including a designated area close to the unit which is comfortable, quiet and private, incorporates both washing and sleeping facilities and where the spiritual needs of the family can be expressed.

(10) An environment to meet the needs and requirements of the nurse will be available, for example sufficient bed area space for staff to work safely while still accommodating the family.

4. PROFESSIONAL PRACTICE

(1) The unit-based nurse makes an initial and ongoing assessment of the following.

(a) The structure of the family unit, the relationships and interactions within this, and the key member of the family preferably identified by the patient.

(b) The social circumstances of the family.

(c) The family's cultural, religious and spiritual needs and beliefs.

(d) The family's previous experience of critical illness.

(e) The family's knowledge and understanding of the patient's illness, prognosis and the possible outcomes of treatment.

(e) The family's physical, psychological and social needs including their needs for information and for maintenance of hope.

(f) The family's emotional and physical reactions.

(g) The family's thoughts and feelings related to the decisions made about the patient's care.

(2) The unit-based nurse analyses the assessment and then plans and implements care in conjunction with the patient, family and other members of the multidisciplinary team.

(a) The nurse liaises with the ward staff and the patient where possible to identify the family as defined by the patient.

(b) The nurse creates time to offer the family information, in a calm and confident manner, honestly and openly, in language understandable to the family and allowing an opportunity for questions.

(c) The nurse liaises with medical colleagues to ensure that families are offered continued information related to the patient's condition and progress.

(d) The nurse spends time establishing rapport and trust with the family and offers support tailored to the family's changing needs.

(e) The nurse provides individualized and sensitive comfort to the family where appropriate – for example by the use of touch.

(f) The nurse recognizes the family's own support network and facilitates this where appropriate.

(g) The nurse fosters a positive but realistic attitude towards the situation in order to fulfil the family's needs for the maintenance of hope.

(h) The nurse actively involves the family in care according to family wishes. This may involve:

- encouraging family members to express their concerns/wishes/opinions
- listening and valuing family wishes
- incorporating family preferences into care where possible and appropriate
- involving family members in practical care.

(i) The nurse ensures that the family's practical needs are met. This may involve:

- encouraging the family to meet their own needs
- liaising with the Accommodation Officer to ensure access to a room
- liaising with social services if the family has financial concerns
- accommodating religious, cultural and spiritual needs where possible and liaising with the chaplain
- ensuring the family has opportunities and facilities to meet their hygiene and dietary needs.

(j) The nurse treats the patient with respect, demonstrating that the patient is cared for and that the staff are interested in and committed to that care (for example by approaching/addressing an unconscious patient as though he or she was able to respond).

(k) The nurse facilitates communication between the patient and family if necessary, encouraging the family to talk with the patient.

(l) The nurse ensures that the family are aware that it is acceptable not to stay with the patient.

(m) The nurse creates an environment where social interaction for the family is possible.

(4) The unit-based nurse monitors and evaluates the effectiveness of care as in (1) and the appropriateness of interventions to meet individual needs.

(5) The unit-based nurse will identify the need to refer the family to other members if the multidisciplinary team, will act where necessary as co-ordinator of the multidisciplinary team and will communicate appropriate information.

(6) The unit-based nurse will facilitate continuity of care on transfer consulting with the ward staff and senior nursing staff where indicated.

(7) The unit-based nurse documents accurately all aspects of professional practice.

5. OUTCOMES

(1) The family report that there was an open and supportive environment and that they were involved in and informed about both patient care and the decision making process to a degree that they determined. They also feel that their needs for education and for emotional and practical support were met.

(2) The nurse considers that he or she had access to the resources listed and was able to follow the described professional practice. The nurse also reports that the family were involved in and informed about both patient care and the decision making process to a degree that the family determined, and that their needs for education and practical and emotional support were met.

(3) The documentation system will show that resources were used and professional practice followed to provide an open and supportive environment and that the family were involved in and informed about both patient care and the decision making process to a degree that they determined. There will be evidence that the patient and family's need for education and for emotional and practical support were met.

REFERENCES

Brawlin, J., Rook, J. and Sills, G. (1982) Families in crisis: the impact of trauma. *Critical Care Quarterly*, Dec. 38–46.

Breu, C. & Dracup, K. (1978) Helping the spouses of critically ill patients. *American Journal of Nursing*, Jan. 50–53.

Coulter, M. (1988) The needs of family members of patients in intensive care units. *Intensive Care Nursing*, **5**, 4–10.

Daley, L. (1984) The perceived immediate needs of families with relatives in the intensive care setting. *Heart and Lung*, **13(2)**, 231–7.

Green, C. (1982) Assessment of family stress. *Journal of Advanced Nursing*, **7**, 11–17.

Molter, N. & Captain, R. (1979) Needs of relatives of critically ill patients – a descriptive study. *Heart and Lung*, **8(2)**, 332–9.

Stillwell, S. B. (1984) Importance of visiting needs as perceived by family members of patients in the intensive care unit. *Heart and Lung*, **15(3)**, 238–42.

CARE OF PATIENTS EXPERIENCING FATIGUE

1. STANDARD STATEMENT

The nursing care of patients who are experiencing fatigue is directed towards supportive measures to maintain optimum individual activity, assisting them to conserve energy, and promoting adjustment/adaption.

2. RATIONALE

Fatigue is a condition characterized by subjective feelings of generalized weariness, exhaustion, and lack of energy resulting from the prolonged stress that is directly or indirectly attributable to the disease process (Aistars, 1987). Fatigue is a universal experience and generally, when a healthy person is fatigued, rest will completely restore that person to their previous level of functioning (Piper et al., 1987, Aistars, 1987).

Acute fatigue is perceived as normal or expected tiredness and symptoms are usually localized to a specific body region. It has a rapid onset and a short duration (days or weeks), appears intermittently and serves a protective function (Riddle, 1982, Piper, 1986). In contrast chronic fatigue is perceived as abnormal or excessive tiredness, tends to involve the whole body and no longer serves a protective function (Cameron, 1973, Poteliakhoff, 1981). Chronic fatigue has been noted as a common and disruptive symptom for individuals with cancer, especially those who are actively undergoing treatment and those with advanced disease (Aistars, 1987). Fatigue can then affect a person's wellbeing, interfere with his or her activities and, ultimately, can have an impact on quality of life.

The actual mechanisms that cause fatigue have not yet been conclusively determined (Piper et al., 1987). Aistars (1987) suggests that prolonged stress is the main cause of chronic fatigue in cancer patients. Whereas Holmes (1988, 1990) states that fatigue arises for two reasons. Firstly, energy demand is increased both by the processes involved in the malignancy itself and by the need for increased anabolism necessary to repair damage to normal cells. Secondly, treatment results in cellular destruction which in turn is associated with the release of both cellular debris and waste products into the circulation. The literature illustrates a wide variety of contributing factors including treatment and disease patterns, sleep and wake patterns, the accumulation of metabolites, psychological and social patterns, etc.

Nursing interventions span the entire treatment continuum, from preventing chronic fatigue (Piper, 1988, Kellum, 1985), screening those at high risk and tailoring therapies to fit different causes and individuals. Nursing assessment needs to consider that the characteristic signs and symptoms vary according to primary cause of lethargy and fatigue (Piper et al., 1989). The nursing management of lethargy and fatigue can be summarized by three strategies (Piper et al., 1989):

- Energy conservation (e.g. delegation, energy conservation methods)
- Effective energy utilization (e.g. prioritizing and pacing activities)
- Energy restoration (e.g. efforts to conserve strength, enhancing nutritional status, reducing the impact of stressors).

Through a holistic, multidisciplinary approach nursing care aims to promote the patient's adaption and adjustment to this condition.

3. RESOURCES

(1) The unit-based nurse will have a baseline knowledge of the following.

(a) The mechanisms and causes of fatigue.
(b) Cell physiology and the cell cycle.
(c) The influences of the following on fatigue:

- cancer and/or its treatment
- symptoms such as pain, dyspnoea, etc.
- psychological factors such as depression
- environmental factors such as noise, temperature, etc.
- social factors such as recent life events, perceived social support
- circadian rhythms
- activity/rest patterns
- sleep/wake patterns
- haematological values.

(d) The physical signs and symptoms of fatigue.
(e) The potential physical problems associated with fatigue (e.g. impaired nutritional status, decreased exercise tolerance, muscle wastage, increased pain, chest infection, etc.).
(f) The psychological impact of fatigue (e.g. lowered mood, feelings of guilt for not being more active, demotivation).
(g) The implications of fatigue on the patient's social, leisure and work activities (e.g. inability to work, reduced social contact) and the effects on the patient's emotional and family relationships.
(h) Pharmacological/non-pharmacological interventions available for amelioration (e.g. steroids, vitamins, dietary supplements, blood products, etc.).
(i) Current research and trends in the management of fatigue, and their implications for both the patient and family and for related nursing care.

(2) The unit-based nurse will have baseline skills in:

(a) Communication – to assess the patient's needs and to determine appropriate times for care.
(b) Teaching – to provide individualized information to the patient and family about the reasons for fatigue, and to offer advice on ways in which to conserve energy.
(c) Practical techniques – to use both pharmacological and non-pharmacological agents in the management of fatigue, and to assist the patient with activities of daily living.

(3) The unit-based nurse will have access to ongoing education and support. The clinical nurse specialist/unit manager will organize supervision, and unit-based teaching sessions, where necessary.

(4) The clinical nurse specialist/unit manager is expected to have detailed knowledge as listed in (1) and skills as in (2). Where the problem has specific management issues/ difficulties, or has become persistent and intractable, a clinical nurse specialist/unit manager with specialist knowledge and skills may be identified to act as a consultant for advice and support.

(5) Other members of the multidisciplinary team will be available to act as a resource or source of referral to the patient, family and nurse including the dietitian, physiotherapist, occupational therapist and psychological care team.

(6) There will be a range of equipment available to the patient, family and nurse – for example, exercise equipment (e.g. an exercise bicycle), diversional/recreational

activities (e.g. a television and radio), complementary therapies, comfortable beds and bedding, and chairs.

(7) The nurse will have access to current written information and research.

(8) An environment suitable to the patient's individual needs will be available, for example there should be a flexible ward routine which considers patients' needs for quiet, rest and sleep.

(9) An environment to met the requirements of the nurse will be available.

4. PROFESSIONAL PRACTICE

(1) The unit-based nurse makes an initial and ongoing assessment of the following.

   (a) The pattern of fatigue (e.g. onset, duration, intensity).
   (b) The patient's prior experience of fatigue.
   (c) The patient's current or past coping strategies related to fatigue.
   (d) The presence of factors contributing to the exacerbation or alleviation of fatigue.
   (e) The patient's general physical condition and nutritional status including the presence of any signs and symptoms of fatigue.
   (f) The patient's normal pattern of daily activity, the patient's job and work environment, leisure and social activities and the impact of fatigue on these.
   (g) The patient and family's understanding and their needs for information, support and education about the causes and management of fatigue.
   (h) The family's willingness, ability and need to participate in the care of the patient.

(2) The unit-based nurse plans and implements care in conjunction with the patient, family and other members of the multidisciplinary team.

   (a) The nurse assists the patient to adjust/adapt his or her activity and lifestyle as appropriate.
   (b) The nurse co-ordinates care in order to minimize unnecessary disruption for the patient and to assist the patient to conserve energy.
   (c) The nurse offers a variety of relaxation strategies/techniques and discusses these with the patient and family to determine which methods are the most suited to the individual.
   (d) The nurse works in conjunction with the patient and family to minimize factors that are known to exacerbate the patient's fatigue.
   (e) The patient is encouraged to use his or her own methods/strategies of relieving lethargy and fatigue where appropriate, and the nurse facilitates these wherever possible.
   (f) The nurse encourages an adequate nutritional input liaising with the dietitian as necessary.
   (g) The nurse administers pharmacological and non-pharmacological agents as necessary, liaising with the medical staff to ensure optimum symptom relief.
   (h) The nurse promotes an environment to facilitate sleep and rest and recognizes the patient's needs for peace and quiet.
   (i) Diversional activities are offered to the patient as appropriate.
   (j) If the patient is to undergo either chemotherapy or radiotherapy, he or she is offered information relating to the usual temporary nature of fatigue and when during the course of treatment it is most likely to occur.
   (k) The nurse offers the patient and family information, support and reassurance

tailored to their individual and changing needs. The patient is supported if he or she wishes not to see visitors and reassured if, due to tiredness, feelings of irritability and anger with the family are experienced.

(l) The family are advised about the timing of visits related to the pattern of the patient's lethargy and fatigue and their needs for rest. The family are also involved (wherever appropriate) in the care of the patient according to their individual preferences.

(3) The unit-based nurse monitors and evaluates the effectiveness of care as in (1) and the appropriateness of interventions to meet individual needs.

(4) The unit-based nurse will identify the need to refer the patient to other members of the multidisciplinary team, will act where necessary as co-ordinator of the multidisciplinary team liaising the timing of interventions/treatments, and will communicate appropriate information.

(5) The unit-based nurse will facilitate continuity of care following discharge/transfer, consulting with the community liaison nurse where indicated.

(6) The unit-based nurse documents accurately all aspects of professional practice.

5. OUTCOMES

(1) The patient and family report that they were able to adjust/adapt to fatigue and that the patient maintained an optimum individual activity. They also report that their needs for education and for emotional and practical support were met.

(2) The nurse considers that he or she had access to the resources as listed and was able to follow the described professional practice. The nurse considers that he or she was able to facilitate the patient's ability to conserve energy, maintain an optimum level of individual activity and adjust or adapt to fatigue, and that the patient and family's needs for education and for emotional and practical support were met.

(3) The documentation system will show evidence that resources were used and professional practice followed to assist the patient to conserve energy, to maintain their optimum individual activity and to adapt or adjust to this problem. There will also be evidence that the patient and family's needs for education and for emotional and practical support were met.

REFERENCES

Aistars, J. (1987) Fatigue in the cancer patient: a conceptual approach to a clinical problem. *Oncology Nursing Forum*, **14(6)**, 25–30.

Cameron, C. (1973) A theory of fatigue. *Ergonomics*, **16(5)**, 633–48.

Holmes, S. (1988) *Radiotherapy*. Lisa Sainsbury Foundation/Austen Cornish, London.

Holmes, S. (1990) *Cancer Chemotherapy*. Lisa Sainsbury Foundation/Austen Cornish, London.

Kellum, M. D. (1985) Fatigue. In *Signs and Symptoms in Nursing: Interpretation and Management*. (Ed. by M. M. Jacobs & W. Feels), pp. 103–18. J.B. Lippincott, Philadelphia.

Piper, B. F. (1986) Fatigue. In *Pathophysiological Phenomena in Nursing: Human Responses to Illness*. (Ed. by V. K. Carrieri, A. M. Lindsey, & C. W. West), pp. 219–34. W.B. Saunders, Philadelphia.

Piper, B. F. (1988) Fatigue in cancer patients: current perspectives on measurement and management. In *Nursing Management of Common Problems. Monograph from the Fifth International Conference on Cancer Nursing*, pp. 24–36. American Cancer Society, New York.

Piper, B. F., Lindsey, A. M. & Dodd, M. J. (1987) Fatigue mechanisms in cancer patients: developing nursing theory. *Oncology Nursing Forum*, **14(6)**, 17–23.

Piper B. F., Rieger, L. B., Brophy, L., Haveber, D., Hood, L. E., Lyver, A. & Sharp, E. (1989) Recent advances in the management of biotherapy-related side effects: fatigue. *Oncology Nursing Forum*, **16(6)**, supplement, 27–34

Poteliakhoff, A. (1981) Adrenocortical activity and some clinical findings in acute and chronic fatigue. *Journal of Bychosomatic Research*, **25(2)**, 91–5.

Riddle, P. K. (1982) Chronic fatigue and women: a description and suggested treatment. *Women and Health*, **7(1)**, 37–47.

NURSING

CARE OF PATIENTS WITH FUNGATING AND ULCERATING MALIGNANT LESIONS

1. STANDARD STATEMENT

The nursing care of patients with fungating and ulcerating malignant lesions is directed towards the minimization of pain, infection, bleeding and odour, and the promotion of an optimal level of comfort for each patient.

2. RATIONALE

A fungating lesion is an additional proliferation of abnormal cellular activity. An ulcerative lesion is an open, eroding, crater type wound. Although fungation and ulceration occur most commonly in breast cancer (Denton, 1989), it may also occur in such sites as the neck, axillae or groin (via lymph node metastases), or the vagina or rectum (via mucous membranes). Although the incidence of fungating and ulcerative lesions appears to have decreased, the potential impact on quality of life remains enormous. Therefore, nursing care which minimizes the impact on quality of life is imperative.

Any underlying factors which might influence wound healing should be noted and appropriate action initiated. The wound should be measured and described, noting the main problems that it causes the patient (Morrison, 1987). The ideal aim is the complete healing of the lesion through either local or systematic treatment (Rosenberg, 1977, Bell, 1983). When such treatments are inappropriate or unsuccessful, then care is directed towards minimization of pain, infection, bleeding and odour (Foltz, 1980). Treatment should be realistic and acceptable to the patient and carers. If the treatment does not promote quality of life and a sense of wellbeing, then it should be changed. Few treatments are absolute. The primary aim should be to promote comfort.

An informed and considered choice regarding the use of conventional and non-conventional topical agents and dressings is as pertinent to the nursing management of malignant lesions as it is to that of other wound types (Butler, 1985, Leaper, 1986). Awareness of, and sensitivity to, the psychological problems that the patient with a malignant lesion may be experiencing is equally important as the control of physical symptoms (Bennet, 1985). This highlights the need to treat not only the wound, but the patient as a whole.

3. RESOURCES

(1) The unit-based nurse will have baseline knowledge of the following.

    (a) Factors leading to malignant fungating lesions (i.e. cancer and its treatment).

    (b) Theory and research on wound healing and management with particular reference to malignant fungating lesions and the appropriate application of cleansing agents and dressings.

    (c) Factors influencing wound healing and progression including nutrition, drug therapies (e.g. steroids), side effects of radiotherapy and chemotherapy, disease progression.

    (d) The physical and psychological impact of malignant fungating lesions on the patient, including pain, odour, altered body image, depression, etc.

    (e) The potential complications associated with particular wound sites (e.g. haemorrhage due to erosion of a major blood vessel) and the action to be taken should they occur.

    (f) The agents available for the management of malignant fungating lesions including systemic agents (e.g. antibiotics), local cleansing agents and dressings and their appropriate research based use(s).

(2) The unit-based nurse will have baseline skills in:

    (a) Communication – to assess psychological impact of the wound and to provide sensitive and individualized support.
    (b) Teaching – to offer the patient and family education related to the care of the wound.
    (c) Practical techniques – such as carrying out aseptic dressing changes.

(3) The unit-based nurse will have access to ongoing education and support. The clinical nurse specialist/unit manager will organize supervision, and unit-based teaching sessions, where necessary.

(4) The clinical nurse specialist/unit manager is expected to have detailed knowledge as listed in (1) and skills as in (2). Where the problem has specific management issues/difficulties or has become persistent and intractable a clinical nurse specialist/unit manager with specialist knowledge and skills may be identified to act as a consultant for advice and support.

(5) Other members of the multidisciplinary team will be available to act as a source of referral or resource to the patient, family and nurse, including relevant clinical nurse specialists, psychological support team, therapeutic massage specialist etc.

(6) There will be a range of specialist equipment and therapeutic agents available for the management of malignant fungating lesions. This should minimally include debriding and cleansing agents and a range of dressings which are known to be effective.

(7) Written information about dressings and treatments will be available for the patient, family and nurse.

(8) An environment suitable for the patient's individual needs will be available (e.g. ensuring privacy, minimizing odours etc.).

(9) An environment suitable for the needs of the nurse will be available (e.g. access to a clean treatment room to prepare dressing trolley).

4. PROFESSIONAL PRACTICE

(1) The unit-based nurse makes an initial and ongoing assessment of the following.

    (a) The previous history of the lesion including how long the patient has had the lesion, previous treatments used and their effectiveness etc.
    (b) The physical appearance of the lesion including its diameter, depth, colour and odour. (The lesion may be photographed as part of this assessment.)
    (c) Any actual or potential complications – for example, by swabbing the lesion to check for infection, observing the site of the lesion to check for risk of bleeding.
    (d) Factors which may exacerbate the condition of the lesion, including disease progression, previous radiotherapy, poor nutritional status certain pharmacological therapies, other co-existing illness, etc.
    (e) Physical symptoms associated with the lesion, such as pain, bleeding, infection or odour.
    (f) The psychological impact of having a malignant fungating lesion – for example, avoidance of others, altered body image, depression.
    (g) The patient's home situation in order to establish whether support will be required in coping with the wound at home (where appropriate).

(2) The unit-based nurse plans and implements care in conjunction with the patient, family and other members of the multidisciplinary team.

(a) The nurse attempts to minimize the symptoms associated with the lesion and promote comfort.
(b) The patient is provided with adequate pain relief (according to his or her individual requirements), particularly prior to changes of dressing, and the nurse liaises with medical staff to ensure optimum symptom control.
(c) The nurse cleans the wound and changes the dressing as often as is appropriate taking into account the requirements of the wound, the dressing used and individual patient wishes.
(d) The nurse offers the patient assistance to adapt to any limitations imposed by the type and site of the wound (e.g. restricted mobility, need for careful positioning, use of aids).
(e) The nurse offers individualized psychological support for the patient and family.
(f) Where appropriate, the nurse teaches the patient and/or family to care for the wound.

(4) The unit-based nurse monitors and evaluates the effectiveness of care as in (1) and the appropriateness of interventions to meet individual needs.

(5) The unit-based nurse identifies the need to refer the patient to other members of the multidisciplinary team, acts where necessary as a co-ordinator of the multidisciplinary team, and communicates appropriate information.

(6) The unit-based nurse facilitates continuity of care following discharge/transfer consulting with the community liaison nurse where indicated and ensuring that the patient and/or family have a contact name or number for follow-up advice and support.

(7) The unit-based nurse documents accurately all aspects of professional practice.

5. OUTCOMES

(1) The patient and family report that the symptoms associated with the malignant lesion are reduced to a minimum, providing an acceptable level of comfort. They will also feel that their needs for education and for emotional and practical support were met.

(2) The nurse considers that he or she had access to the resources as listed and was able to follow the described professional practice. The nurse also feels that the symptoms associated with the patient's malignant lesion were reduced to a minimum, providing a level of comfort acceptable to the individual patient.

(3) The documentation system will show evidence that resources were used and professional practice followed to minimize the pain, infection, bleeding and odour associated with the malignant lesion and promote a level of comfort acceptable to the individual patient. There will also be evidence that the patient and family's needs for education and for emotional and practical support were met.

REFERENCES

Bell, M. (1983) Fungating carcinoma of the breast. *Nursing Times*, **79(21)**, 60–1.
Bennet, M. (1985) As normal a life as possible. *Community Outlook*, **81(7)**, 35–8.

Butler, G. A. (1985) Desloughing agents at work. *Nursing Mirror*, **160(13)**, 29.

Denton, S. (1989) In *Oncology for Nurses and Health Professionals*, Vol. 3, 2nd edn (Ed. by R. Tiffany), pp. 309–339. Harper & Row, London.

Foltz, A. T. (1980) Nursing care of ulcerated lesions. *Oncology Nursing Forum*, **7(2)**, 8–13.

Leaper, D. (1986) Antiseptics and their effect on the healing tissue. *Nursing Times*, **82(22)**, 45–7.

Morrison, M. J. (1987) Factsheet – Wound management: Part 2. *Professional Nurse*, September 1987 (Insert).

Rosenberg, F. W. (1977) Cutaneous manifestations of internal malignancy. *Cutis*, **20(2)**, 227–34.

NURSING

CARE OF PATIENTS WHO ARE INCONTINENT OF URINE

1. STANDARD STATEMENT

The nursing care of patients who are incontinent of urine is directed towards promoting continence wherever possible by thorough assessment and individualized care. Nursing care is also directed towards facilitating adaption to this problem in order to maintain self-esteem and enabling patients to integrate wherever possible the management of urinary incontinence into their everyday lives. Patients and their families will be offered comprehensive information and support.

2. RATIONALE

Incontinence is one of the most distressing forms of disablement. The experience of incontinence for sufferers can be devastating, involving loss of self-esteem, embarrassment and the effective cessation of social activities. The prevalence of incontinence is often vastly underestimated. It occurs because of an involuntary loss of urine which has become a social or hygiene problem. This may result from a variety of conditions including congenital abnormalities, urinary fistula, carcinoma of the prostate, bladder neck obstruction and urethral stricture. Incontinence is a symptom of an underlying disorder and not an illness itself.

Nurses play a key role both in the identification of the problem and in the provision of advice and support for incontinent individuals and their family or carers. To maximize individualized patient care it is essential for nurses to have an in-depth knowledge of the current trends and the research tested treatments which are available, thus allowing nurses to initiate appropriate interventions wherever possible.

As advocated by Norton (1986), nurses have a responsibility to patients and their families to utilize the best available expertise in providing care, both for the promotion of continence and in fostering a positive approach towards incontinence among carers.

3. RESOURCES

(1) The unit-based nurse will have a baseline knowledge of the following.

  (a) The anatomy and physiology of the genito-urinary tract and the physiology of micturition.
  (b) The causes of urinary incontinence including cancer and/or its treatment (e.g. urinary tract infection, trauma to the pelvic floor muscles, etc.)
  (c) Other physical factors influencing urinary incontinence (e.g. Parkinsons disease, diabetes, etc.)
  (d) The influences of psychological factors such as anxiety on incontinence.
  (e) The physical implications of urinary incontinence for a patient.
  (f) The psychological impact of urinary incontinence on the patient (e.g. lowered self-esteem).
  (g) The possible impact of urinary incontinence on the patient's personal relationships, work and leisure activities (e.g. decreased social contact).
  (h) The implications of urinary incontinence on the patient's sexuality and sexual activity.
  (i) The aids and equipment available for the management of urinary incontinence and their indications for use.
  (j) Current research and trends in the management of urinary incontinence, and their implications for both the patient and family and for related nursing care.

(2) The unit-based nurse will have baseline skills in:

(a) Communication – to convey a sensitive and empathetic attitude, to minimize feelings of embarrassment and to provide information and support. Also, observational skills to assess patient's needs – particularly when patients use differing language or terms for incontinence.

(b) Teaching – to educate the patient and family about self-catheterization, pelvic floor exercises etc.

(c) Practical techniques – for example, to adapt and use aids and equipment available for the management of urinary incontinence.

(3) The unit-based nurse will have access to ongoing education and support. The clinical nurse specialist/unit manager will organize supervision, and unit-based teaching sessions, where necessary.

(4) The clinical nurse specialist (stoma care/incontinence) will have a detailed knowledge as listed in (1) in particular the current trends and developments in the management of incontinence and the availability of equipment and resources. The clinical nurse specialist will also have a wider range of teaching and practical skills, and advanced communication skills in order to provide in depth assessment and care. He or she will be available to act as a resource or source of referral for the patient, family and nurse.

The clinical nurse specialist (stoma care/incontinence) will also co-ordinate a core group of health care professionals with an interest in incontinence. The aims of the group, which is a member of The Continence Advisors Association, are to discuss and investigate the causes of incontinence and to formulate a systematic approach to the assessment and management of incontinence.

(5) Other members of the multidisciplinary team will be available to act as a resource or source of referral to the patient, family and nurse including medical staff, occupational therapists, physiotherapists and the appliance officer.

(6) There will be a range of equipment available to the patient, family and nurse (e.g. incontinence pads, sheaths, etc.)

(7) The nurse will have access to current written information and research concerning the care of patients who are incontinent of urine.

(8) Written information will be available to the patient and family including information booklets about intermittent self-catherization and all aspects of incontinence, information about support groups outside the hospital (e.g. the Urostomy Association), and information about the availability of aids and equipment.

(9) An environment suitable to the patient's individual needs will be available (e.g. ensuring privacy).

(10) An environment to meet the needs/requirements of the nurse – including access to a single room for patient interviews where appropriate – will be available.

4. PROFESSIONAL PRACTICE

(1) The unit-based nurse makes an initial and ongoing assessment of the following.

(a) The patient's pattern of micturition and their urinary symptoms including whether they experience frequency and/or nocturia, the nature of their urine stream etc.

(b) The patient's bowel function and any current changes.

(c) The patient's level of mobility.

(d) The patient's current/previous medications.

(e) The emotional response of the patient (and family) to the problem of urinary incontinence – for example, feelings of embarrassment and low self-esteem.

(f) The patient's home environment (e.g. accessibility of toilet facilities), the family structure and relationships and the patient's level of emotional support.

(g) The patient's job and work environment, leisure and social activities and the impact of incontinence on these (e.g. reduced social contact due to fears of incontinence, increased laundry demands, etc.)

(h) The patient and family's ability (e.g. their visual acuity and their manual dexterity) and willingness to participate in the management of urinary incontinence.

(i) The patient and family's needs for information, support and education about both the urinary incontinence and the proposed plan of treatment.

(2) The unit-based nurse analyses the assessment and liaises with medical colleagues in order to identify wherever possible the cause(s) of the urinary incontinence.

(3) The unit-based nurse plans and implements care in conjunction with the patient, family and other members of the multidisciplinary team.

(a) The nurse initiates strategies/methods to relieve the cause(s) of the urinary incontinence wherever possible (e.g. teaching pelvic floor exercises, designing individualized toilet training programmes, ensuring constipation is relieved or a urinary tract infection is treated, etc.)

(b) The nurse provides supportive measures appropriate to the cause of incontinence. For example, if the patient is experiencing radiation cystitis the nurse encourages oral fluids, educates the patient about skin care and liaises with medical colleagues to ensure that pain relief is provided.

(c) Where appropriate, the nurse discusses with the patient and family long term management of the problem – for example permanent catherization if the cause is spinal cord compression, or intermittent self-catherization if the patient has a stricture, etc.

(d) The nurse offers the patient and family information and support tailored to their individual and changing needs.

(e) The nurse ensures that the patient has the necessary aids and equipment, liaising with the occupational therapist (e.g. for a raised toilet seat) and with the appliance officer and/or district nurse (e.g. for pads) as appropriate.

(f) The nurse offers specific information regarding the management of urinary incontinence in the patient's home environment including where to obtain and how to dispose of equipment.

(g) The patient and family are offered information on the statutory and voluntary services available in the community.

(h) The nurse ensures wherever possible that the patient has been referred to a continence advisor for follow-up in the community.

(4) The unit-based nurse monitors and evaluates the effectiveness of care as in (1) and the appropriateness of interventions to meet individual needs.

(5) The unit-based nurse will identify the need to refer the patient to other members if the multidisciplinary team, will act where necessary as co-ordinator of the multidisciplinary team and will communicate appropriate information.

(6) The unit-based nurse will facilitate continuity of care on discharge/transfer, consulting with the community liaison nurse where indicated, and ensuring that the patient and/or family have a contact name or number for follow-up advice and support.

(7) The unit-based nurse documents accurately all aspects of professional practice.

5. OUTCOMES

(1) The patient and family feel that they were able to discuss urinary incontinence and that they were able to integrate wherever possible the management of the problem into their everyday lives. They also feel that their needs for education and for emotional and practical support were met.

(2) The nurse considers that he or she had access to the resources as listed and was able to follow the described professional practice. The nurse also considers that, through the provision of education, information and support he or she was able to promote continence, create an opportunity where the patient felt able to discuss urinary incontinence and assist the patient to integrate its management into her or his everyday life.

(3) The documentation system will show evidence that resources were used and professional practice followed to promote continence, to create an environment where the patient felt able to discuss incontinence and to assist the patient to integrate the management of urinary incontinence into everyday life. There will also be evidence that the patient and family's needs for education and for emotional and practical support were met.

REFERENCES

Norton, C. (1986) *Nursing for Continence*. Beaconsfield Publishers, Beaconsfield.

CARE OF PATIENTS WHO ARE NAUSEATED AND VOMITING

1. STANDARD STATEMENT

The nursing care of patients who experience nausea and vomiting is directed towards the control and relief of these symptoms. Care is also directed towards enhancing physiological and psychological wellbeing, and preventing or minimizing dehydration, weight loss and malnutrition.

2. RATIONALE

Within the context of cancer nursing, nausea and vomiting are common problems. Most literature focusses on chemotherapy induced nausea and vomiting rather than that induced by radiotherapy or the disease itself. In the context of chemotherapy, nausea and vomiting are reputed to be two of the most disruptive side-effects associated with this treatment (Richardson, 1991). Currently nausea and vomiting are poorly managed (Richardson, 1989) and have been identified by cancer patients (Todres & Wojtiuck, 1979, Kennedy et al., 1981, Needleman, 1987), oncologists (Frytal & Moertel, 1981) and oncology nurses (Oberst, 1978, Degner et al., 1987, Pritchard & Speechley, 1989) as a major concern.

The phenomenon of nausea and vomiting is a highly sophisticated protective mechanism developed as part of the body's homeostatic systems helping to rid the body of noxious substances and stimuli. It is generally accepted that there are three independent stages — nausea, retching and vomiting, which usually occur in tandem, but which should not be considered as part of a single symptom complex (Richardson, 1989). Nausea is the subjective awareness of the need to vomit which generally, but not always, culminates in vomiting. Retching consists of rhythmic, laboured spasmodic movements involving the diaphragm, chest wall and abdominal muscles. Retching usually precedes or alternates with vomiting and forces the intestinal contents upwards. Vomiting is the involuntary reflex causing the forceful expulsion of the contents of the stomach and intestine through the mouth and nose. Vomiting is controlled by the vomiting centre and stimulation may occur from a number of sources including the chemotrigger zone, the periphery and central nervous systems (Richardson, 1989).

The physical consequences of nausea and vomiting for the patient can be severe, for example, patients may be unable to eat properly which may lead to nutritional deficits, dehydration, electrolyte imbalances, fatigue and weakness. Nausea and vomiting may range from a tolerable mild discomfort to serious complications (Richardson, 1991), for example gastrointestinal trauma (Enck, 1977). These stresses are compounded by the psychological stresses. Exhaustion can lead to a disruption in lifestyle, and anxiety and depression may occur (Richardson, 1991). Studies have highlighted that many patients come to view treatment and the resulting discomfort as worse than the disease itself and are reluctant to subject themselves to repeated courses of treatment (e.g. Stroudermire et al., 1984, Lazlo & Lucus, 1981).

Numerous studies have described the many pharmacological and behavioural strategies to lessen nausea and vomiting (e.g. Yasko, 1985, Wickham, 1989) whereas there is a dearth of literature related to the performance and effectiveness of self-care activities in cancer patients to control nausea and vomiting. Self-care has been suggested as a means of promoting more successful symptom control. Preliminary studies by Richardson (1991) and Li-Huan Lo (1990), however, have begun to explore the self-care behaviours used by chemotherapy patients.

Patients should not have to endure severe unrelenting nausea and vomiting for palliation, control or cure of cancer (Wickham, 1989). Nurses' concern for symptom control must be of prime importance as nurses have a major role in the management of nausea and vomiting. Nursing care must be based on detailed individualized assessment that includes the physical and psychological impact of nausea and vomiting for the patient and any self-care activities that the patient participates in such as sleep and diversional activities and modification of food and fluid intake. The planning and implementation of care must also account for the patient's disease status and the treatment (if any) being administered.

3. RESOURCES

(1) The unit-based nurse will have baseline knowledge of the following.

- (a) The physiology of nausea and vomiting.
- (b) The anatomy and physiology of the gastrointestinal tract.
- (c) The causes of nausea and vomiting related to cancer and/or its treatment.
- (d) Factors contributing to the exacerbation of nausea and vomiting (e.g. anxiety, pain, psychological triggers causing anticipatory nausea and vomiting, emetic stimuli such as food odours).
- (e) Pharmacological methods used in the control/relief of nausea and vomiting (e.g. anti-emetics – their actions, efficacy and side-effects).
- (f) Non-pharmacological methods available for the control/relief of nausea and vomiting (e.g. self-care strategies, relaxation techniques, distraction, aromatherapy, acupuncture, seabands, etc.)
- (g) The physical implication of nausea and vomiting on the patient (e.g. weakness and lethargy, dehydration, malnourishment, weight loss, etc.)
- (h) The psychological implications of nausea and vomiting for the patient (e.g. anxiety, low mood, feelings of embarrassment, etc.)
- (i) The implications of nausea and vomiting on the patient's social and work activities (e.g. inability to work, reduced social contact, and the effects on patient's emotional and family relationships).
- (j) Current research and trends in the management of nausea and vomiting, and their implications for both the patient and family and related nursing care.

(2) The unit-based nurse will have baseline skills in:

- (a) Communication – in order to comfort and reassure the patient, to convey a sensitive, empathetic and supportive attitude and to assess the patient's experience of nausea and vomiting.
- (b) Teaching – to educate the patient and family about the methods of controlling/relieving nausea and vomiting.
- (c) Practical techniques – for example, for the appropriate timing of anti-emetics and/or meals, demonstrating relaxation techniques, administering pharmacological therapies, etc.

(3) The unit-based nurse will have access to ongoing education and support. The clinical nurse specialist/unit manager will organize supervision, and unit-based teaching sessions, where necessary.

(4) The clinical nurse specialist/unit manager will have detailed knowledge as listed in (1) and skills as in (2). Where a problem has specific management issues/difficulties or has become persistent and intractable then a clinical nurse specialist/unit manager with specialist knowledge and skills may be identified to act as a consultant for advice and support.

(5) Other members of the multidisciplinary team will be available to act as a resource or source of referral for the patient, family and nurse including the pharmacist, dietitian, medical staff and the psychological care team.

(6) There will be a range of equipment available to the patient, family and nurse including mouthcare equipment, deodorisers, supplementary foodstuffs, audio-visual equipment etc.

(7) Written information will be available to the patient, family and nurse including the patient information booklets on chemotherapy, radiotherapy and on overcoming eating difficulties.

(8) An environment to meet the patient's individual needs will be available, for example location of the patient on the ward in relation to food preparation areas, proximity to bathroom, toilet etc., and privacy wherever possible and desired by the patient.

(9) An environment to meet the needs/requirements of the nurse will be available.

4. PROFESSIONAL PRACTICE

(1) The unit-based nurse makes an initial and ongoing assessment of the following.

(a) The reasons or possible reasons for nausea and vomiting.
(b) The current problem – the timing of the nausea and/or vomiting, its duration and frequency.
(c) The patient's perceptions of the nausea and vomiting as a problem – i.e. what is an acceptable or unacceptable level of nausea and vomiting.
(d) The patient's prior experience of nausea and vomiting associated with cancer and/or its treatment.
(e) The patient's current or past coping or self-care strategies related to nausea and vomiting (e.g. iced water, dry crackers or sleep).
(f) The patient's current/previous medications (e.g. anti-emetics, their dosage and frequency, etc.)
(g) The presence of factors contributing to either the relief or exacerbation of the nausea and vomiting.
(h) The patient's general physical condition including an oral assessment, the condition of the patient's skin, the patient's fluid and nutritional status, etc.
(i) The patient's psychological state (e.g. whether the patient is withdrawn, depressed, etc.)
(j) The patient's home environment, the family structure and relationships, and the patient and family's needs for information, support and education about the causes and management of nausea and vomiting.
(k) The patient's job and work environment, leisure and social activities and the impact of nausea and vomiting on these.
(l) The family's willingness, ability and need to participate in the care of the patient.

(2) The unit-based nurse plans and implements care in conjunction with the patient, family and other members of the multidisciplinary team.

(a) The nurse ensures that symptomatic relief is provided in accordance with individual patient preferences wherever possible, utilizing pharmacological and non-pharmacological methods as appropriate. The nurse liaises with medical staff to ensure optimal symptom relief.

(b) The nurse encourages and facilitates the patient to use his or her own methods of relieving nausea and vomiting where appropriate.

(c) The nurse ensures that factors which are known to exacerbate the patient's nausea and vomiting are alleviated or reduced, and that those known to relieve it are promoted wherever possible.

(d) The nurse promotes patient comfort by, for example, providing oral care and ensuring patient privacy wherever possible.

(e) The nurse encourages an adequate nutritional and fluid intake, liaising with the dietitian and medical staff as necessary.

(f) The nurse ensures that the patient has an opportunity for adequate sleep and rest.

(g) The nurse offers the patient and family information, support and reassurance tailored to their individual and changing needs.

(h) The family are advised about the timing of visits related both to treatment and to the pattern of nausea and vomiting. The family are also involved (wherever appropriate) in the care of the patient according to their individual preferences.

(3) The unit-based nurse monitors and evaluates the effectiveness of care as in (1) and the appropriateness of interventions to meet individual needs.

(4) The unit-based nurse will identify the need to refer the patient to other members of the multidisciplinary team, will act where necessary as a co-ordinator of the multidisciplinary team liaising about the timing of interventions/treatments, and will communicate appropriate information.

(5) The unit-based nurse will facilitate continuity of care following discharge/transfer, consulting with the community liaison nurse where indicated.

(6) The unit-based nurse documents accurately all aspects of professional practice.

5. OUTCOMES

(1) The patient and family feel that nausea and vomiting were controlled/relieved, that environmental needs were met and that the patient's coping and self-care strategies were facilitated and accommodated. They will also feel that their needs for education and for emotional and practical support were met.

(2) The nurse considers that he or she had access to the resources as listed and was able to follow the described professional practice. The nurse also considers that nausea and vomiting were controlled or relieved, and that the patient and family's needs for education and for emotional and practical support were met. The nurse also considers that he or she was able to facilitate and accommodate self-care strategies and that the environmental needs of the patient were met.

(3) The documentation system will show evidence that resources were used and professional practice followed to control or relieve nausea and vomiting. There will also be evidence that the patient and family's needs for education and for emotional and practical support were met.

REFERENCES

Degner, L. *et al.* (1987) Priorities for cancer nursing research. *Cancer Nursing*, **2(4)**, 283–6
Enck, F. (1977) Mallory-Weiss lesion following chemotherapy. *Lancet*, **ii**, 927–8.

Frytal, S. & Moertel, C. (1981) Management of nausea and vomiting in the cancer patient. *Journal of the American Medical Association*, **245**, 393–6.

Kennedy, M., Packard, R., Grant, M. & Padilla, G. (1981) Chemotherapy related nausea and vomiting: a survey to identify problems and interventions. *Oncology Nursing Forum*, **8(1)**, 19–21.

Lazlo, J. & Lucus, V. (1981) Emesis as a critical problem in chemotherapy. *New England Journal of Medicine*, **16**, 948–9.

Li-Huan, Lo. (1990) Assessing breast cancer patients' self care behaviours for nausea and vomiting from chemotherapy. *Oncology Nursing Forum*, **17(2)**, (supplement), 141.

Needleman, R. (1987) Chemotherapy; an overview of nausea and vomiting in the cancer patient. *Association of Associated Occupational Health Nurses*, **35(4)**, 179–82.

Oberst, M. (1978) Priorities in cancer nursing research. *Cancer Nursing*, **1**, 281–90.

Pritchard, A. P. & Speechley, V. (1989) What do nurses know about emesis? *International Cancer News*, **1**, 1.

Richardson, A. (1989) Self care. A study of the behaviours initiated by chemotherapy patients to control nausea and vomiting. Unpublished Msc. Thesis. Kings College, University of London.

Richardson, A. (1991) Theories of self care: their relevance to chemotherapy induced nausea and vomiting. *Journal of Advanced Nursing*, **16**, 671–6.

Stroudermire, A., Contanch, P. & Lazlo, J. (1984) Recent advances in the pharmacologic and behaviourial management of chemotherapy induced emesis. *Archives of Internal Medicine*, **144**, 1029–33.

Todres, R. & Wojtiuck, R. (1979) The cancer patient's view of chemotherapy. *Cancer Nursing*, **2(4)**, 283–6.

Wickham, R. (1989) Managing chemotherapy induced nausea and vomiting: the state of the art. *Oncology Nursing Forum*, **16(4)**, 563–74.

Yasko, J. (1985) Holistic management of nausea and vomiting caused by chemotherapy. *Topics in Clinical Nursing*, **17**, 26–36.

CARE OF PATIENTS AT RISK OF, OR WITH, ORAL COMPLICATIONS

NURSING

1. STANDARD STATEMENT

The nursing care of patients who are at risk of developing oral complications as a result of their disease and/or its treatment is directed towards preventing or minimizing distressing symptoms and reducing the risk of oral infections.

2. RATIONALE

Oral complications are a common problem associated with certain chemotherapeutic agents and head and neck radiotherapy. Stomatitis, mucositis, altered taste and salivatory changes may have significant implications for patients. Patients' sense of wellbeing may be challenged not only by their oral complications but also by the accompanying symptoms – pain, inability to chew, difficulty in opening the mouth and dry mouth (Bersani & Carl, 1983). The potential oral complications make adequate oral intake difficult, if not impossible. In addition, oral effects of treatment combined with treatment related immunosuppression make the mouth a favourite site for ulceration, haemorrhage and infection (Peterson & Sond, 1983). Every such infection is potentially lethal since the damaged mucosa may serve as a port of entry to the bloodstream, leading to septicaemia.

Research has suggested that preventative oral care significantly reduces oral complications of chemotherapy (Beck, 1979) and the incidence of acute peridental infections in patients receiving immunosuppressant therapy (Peterson *et al.*, 1981). Therefore the primary focus of nursing care is thorough assessment and the facilitation of meticulous oral care. If complications do arise, collaboration with medical and dietitian colleagues is imperative to provide prompt treatment and minimization of distressing symptoms.

3. RESOURCES

(1) The unit-based nurse will have knowledge of the following:

    (a) The normal anatomy and physiology (including appearance) of the mouth.

    (b) The potential effects of radiotherapy and chemotherapy on the mouth and their mechanisms of action.

    (c) The correct use of an oral assessment chart.

    (d) The signs of oral complications, including the identification of specific symptoms and infections.

    (e) The action to be taken should particular symptom(s) and/or infection(s) occur.

    (f) The potential complications of oral trauma and infection (e.g. septicaemia), and the implications of these for the patient.

    (g) The pharmacological and non-pharmacological agents available to prevent or treat oral symptoms, and their appropriate application and relative benefits.

    (h) The dietary supplements available for patients with oral problems, and their indications for use.

    (i) Current research and trends in the management of oral complications, and their implications for both the patient and family and for related nursing care.

(2) The unit-based nurse will have baseline skills in:

    (a) Communication – to gain the confidence of the patient and family, to provide sensitive support and information and to facilitate compliance with the oral hygiene regime.

NURSING

(b) Teaching – to teach both the patient and family about the importance and methods of mouth care and about possible complications.

(c) Practical techniques – for example, in observation and recognition of specific oral complications, use of the oral assessment tool and the application of pharmacological and non-pharmacological agents.

(3) The unit-based nurse will have access to ongoing education and support. The clinical nurse specialist/unit manager will organize supervision, and informal unit-based teaching sessions, where necessary.

(4) The clinical nurse specialist/unit manager is expected to have detailed knowledge as listed in (1) and skills as in (2). Where the problem has specific management issues/difficulties or has become persistent and intractable a clinical nurse specialist/unit manager with specialist knowledge and skills may be identified to act as a consultant for advice and support.

(5) Other members of the multidisciplinary team will be available to act as a resource or source of referral to the patient, family and nurse including the clinical nurse specialist (infection control), the oral hygienist, a dentist, pharmacist and the medical team.

(6) There will be a range of specialist equipment available for the prevention/treatment of oral complications, including a torch, mirror, swabs, pharmacological and non-pharmacological agents, etc.

(7) The nurse will have access to current written information and research concerning oral care for patients undergoing chemotherapy/radiotherapy, including the indications and contraindications for the use of pharmacological/non-pharmacological therapies and the hospital policy for protective isolation.

(8) Written information on oral hygiene will be available to the patient and family.

(9) An environment suitable to the patient's individual needs will be available (e.g. ensuring privacy, easy access to toilet and washbasin).

(10) An environment to meet the needs/requirements of the nurse (e.g. having access to a clean treatment area) will be available.

4. PROFESSIONAL PRACTICE

(1) The unit-based nurse makes an initial and ongoing assessment of the following.

(a) Past history of oral problems, either related to previous treatment or other causes.

(b) Past history of oral therapies.

(c) Whether the patient has had pre-admission check-ups by his or her own dentist and the hospital oral hygienist (bone marrow transplant patients only).

(d) The current condition of the patient's mouth – using the oral assessment scale.

(e) The potential oral complications which can be anticipated as a result of treatment(s).

(f) The patient's (and family's) knowledge and understanding of potential oral complications, how these may be prevented or minimized, and their ability and desire to participate in care.

(g) Nutritional status and implications of oral complications.

(h) Psychological impact of actual/potential oral problems on the patient and family.

(2) The unit-based nurse plans and implements care in conjunction with the patient, family and other relevant members of the multidisciplinary team.

    (a) The patient and family are provided with information concerning potential oral problems to ensure understanding and compliance.

    (b) The patient (and family) are offered teaching related to the regime and practical skills of oral care to encourage self-care wherever possible and desirable to the patient.

    (c) Where the patient and family are unable or unwilling to carry out oral care, the nurse assists the patient as necessary.

    (d) The patient is screened for signs of local and systemic complications by observation using the oral assessment scale at least daily and comparing scores and by taking regular swabs (according to unit policy).

    (e) Symptomatic relief (e.g. administering analgesia, offering cold/warm drinks, etc.) is provided in accordance with individual patient preference.

    (f) Where infection is suspected or identified, appropriate treatment is initiated (in conjunction with medical staff).

    (g) The patient and family are offered support and provided with regular information on the condition of the patient's mouth and when they can expect healing to begin.

    (h) The nurse encourages an adequate nutritional and fluid intake (liaising with the dietitian and medical staff as necessary).

(3) The unit-based nurse monitors and evaluates the effectiveness of care as in (1) and the appropriateness of treatments to meet individual needs.

(4) The unit-based nurse will identify the need to refer the patient to other members of the multidisciplinary team, will act where necessary as co-ordinator of the multidisciplinary team and will communicate appropriate information.

(5) The unit-based nurse facilitates continuity of care following discharge/transfer, consulting with the community liaison nurse where indicated.

(6) The unit-based nurse documents accurately all aspects of professional practice.

5. OUTCOMES

(1) The patient and family report that distressing symptoms (and infection) were prevented/minimized. They also feel that their needs for education and for practical and emotional support were met.

(2) The nurse considers that he or she had access to the resources as listed and was able to follow the described professional practice. The nurse reports that distressing symptoms and infection were prevented or minimized. The nurse considers that the patient's and family's needs for education and for practical and emotional support were met.

(3) The documentation system will show evidence that resources were used and professional practice followed ensuring that distressing symptoms and infection were prevented or minimized. There will be evidence that the patient's and family's needs for education and for practical and emotional support were met.

NURSING

REFERENCES

Beck, S. (1979) Impact of a systemic oral care protocol on stomatitis after chemotherapy. *Cancer Nursing*, **2**, 185–99.

Bersani, G. & Carl, W. (1983) Oral care for cancer patients. *American Journal of Nursing*, **83**, 533–6.

Peterson, D. E. *et al.* (1981) Relationship of intensive oral hygiene to systemic complications in acute non-lymphocytic leukaemia patients. *Clinical Research*, **29**, 440A.

Peterson, D. E. & Sond, S. T. (1983) *Oral Complications of Cancer Chemotherapy (Developments in Oncology* Vol. 12). Martinus Nijholf, The Hague.

CARE OF PATIENTS REQUIRING POST-OPERATIVE PAIN CONTROL

1. STANDARD STATEMENT

Nursing care for patients who have surgery is directed towards the provision of individualized pain control to relieve or control post-operative pain.

2. RATIONALE

The treatment of pain after surgery is central to the care of post-operative patients and failure to relieve such pain is morally and ethically unacceptable (Royal College of Surgeons & College of Anaesthetists, 1990). As Liebeskind and Melzack (1987) state 'by any reasonable code freedom from pain should be a basic human right limited only by our knowledge to achieve it'. Numerous studies have shown, however, that many patients experience an unacceptable level of pain after surgery. Cohen (1980), for example, reported that 75% of patients experienced moderate to severe pain following abdominal surgery. Cartwright (1985) demonstrated that nurses' attitudes, beliefs and knowledge about the effectiveness, duration of action and side-effects of analgesia contributed to inadequate pain control. Improper application of both current knowledge and assessment skills by nurses also contribute to inadequate pain management (Bonica, 1980).

Post-operative pain has implications for patients' respiratory function, cardiovascular system, gastrointestinal system and stress response to surgery. Patients may become fatigued and demoralized, and pain after surgery may interfere with sleep in 70% of patients (Royal College of Surgeons & College of Anaesthetists, 1990). As members of the multidisciplinary team, nurses are instrumental in the assessment, management and evaluation of post-operative pain. Through accurate and individualized assessment, for example, the nurse can ensure improved pain management (McCaffrey, 1979).

3. RESOURCES

(1) The unit-based nurse will have a baseline knowledge of the following.

    (a) Theories of pain.

    (b) The methods of administration, action, and side-effects of pharmacological agents used in the management of acute post-operative pain (e.g. analgesics, co-analgesics and anaesthetic agents such as entonox).

    (c) Non-pharmacological interventions used in the management of post-operative pain.

    (d) Pain assessment (taking into account physical, emotional and spiritual components).

    (e) The use of tools for the assessment and recording of pain.

    (f) Physiological and psychological effects of pain.

    (g) The surgery performed and the related anatomy.

    (h) Positioning of the body and support of the wound to reduce pain.

    (i) Up-to-date knowledge of the indications for and correct use of equipment in the management of acute post-operative pain (e.g. intravenous and subcutaneous syringe drivers).

    (j) The factors influencing pain (e.g. anxiety, isolation, insomnia, etc.)

    (k) The current research, trends and developments in post-operative pain relief (e.g. patient-controlled analgesia).

(2) The unit-based nurse will have baseline skills in:

    (a) Communication – to recognize verbal and non-verbal expression of pain, to assess patient's experience of pain and to provide psychological support and information.

    (b) Teaching – for effective education of patient and family of the potential experience of post-operative pain, the need for regular analgesia particularly with reference to post-operative exercise and the actions that the patient can initiate to reduce pain.

    (c) Practical techniques – for example, in drug administration, setting up and using syringe drivers.

(3) The unit-based nurse will have access to ongoing education and support. The clinical nurse specialist/unit manager will organize supervision, and unit-based teaching sessions, where necessary.

(4) Where surgery is a prevelant therapy, the clinical nurse specialist/unit manager will have detailed knowledge as listed in (1) and skills as listed in (2). The clinical nurse specialist/unit manager will provide expert nursing care where the problem has specific management issues/difficulties or has become persistent and intractable. She or he will liaise with other members of the multidisciplinary team to provide all the possible options to control or relieve the pain. She or he also supervises and acts as a resource to ward staff in providing routine post-operative pain care.

(5) Other members of the multidisciplinary team will be available to act as a resource or source of referral to the patient, family and nurse. Such team members include pharmacist, anaesthetist, surgeon, physiotherapist, therapeutic masseur and occupational therapist.

(6) There will be a range of pharmacological and non-pharmacological therapies/aids available including IV pumps, transcutaneous nerve stimulator (TNS) machines, hot and cold packs, lymphoedema pillows and Spenco mattresses and bed cradles.

(7) There will be a range of diversional therapies including televisions, cassette recorders and relaxation tapes.

(8) Written information will be available to the patient and family (e.g. post-operative exercise sheets, information about surgery and treatments).

(9) An environment suitable to the needs of the patient and family (e.g. quiet, with correct temperature and lighting) will be available.

(10) An environment suitable to the needs the of the nurse (e.g. an area to store equipment, privacy for information giving prior to surgery) will be provided.

4. PROFESSIONAL PRACTICE

(1) The unit-based nurse makes a pre-operative assessment of the following.

    (a) The patient's feelings about hospitalization, the patient's expectations of the surgery and the likely post-operative pain.

    (b) The patient's and family's educational needs regarding the surgery and post-operative pain.

(c) The presence of concurrent pains.
(d) The patient's past experience and perceptions of pain.
(e) Current factors influencing pain including anxiety, cultural background, personality.
(f) The patient's level of emotional support.
(g) The patient and family's willingness and ability to be involved in the management of post-operative pain.

(2) The unit-based nurse makes an ongoing post-operative assessment of the following.

(a) The patient's physical experience of surgery and anaesthesia.
(b) The nature, degree, location and duration of pain.
(c) The effectiveness of pharmacological and non-pharmacological interventions.
(d) The patient's and family's psychological response to surgery and pain.
(e) The factors alleviating or exacerbating post-operative pain (e.g. patient positioning, post-operative infection).

(3) The unit-based nurse plans and implements pre-operative care in conjunction with the patient, family and other members of the multidisciplinary team.

(a) The patient and family are offered general information concerning pre-operative preparation and what to expect post-operatively (e.g. wound sites and drains).
(b) The patient and family are offered specific information relating to the sensations the patient is likely to experience post-operatively (including numbness and pain), and the sources of post-operative pain (e.g. drain sites, exercises etc.)
(c) The patient and family are advised on the contribution they can make to the relief of post-operative pain (e.g. requesting analgesia, using relaxation exercises if appropriate, supporting the wound).
(d) The patient and family are provided with an opportunity to ask questions and to discuss their concerns or fears.

(4) The unit-based nurse plans and implements post-operative care in conjunction with the patients, family and other members of the multidisciplinary team.

(a) The patient's pain is assessed.
(b) Pharmacological interventions are initiated at regular intervals and promptly, taking into account individual patient preference wherever possible.
(c) The nurse liaises with medical colleagues to ensure optimal pain relief.
(d) Non-pharmacological interventions are initiated where necessary liaising with the relevant member of the multidisciplinary team as necessary (e.g. physiotherapist, therapeutic masseur).
(e) The nurse ensures that the patient is either pain free or pain relief is initiated prior to potentially painful procedures (e.g. physiotherapy, dressing changes).
(f) The patient and family are offered support and reassurance, and are provided with information on the patient's condition and progress.

(5) The unit-based nurse monitors and evaluates the effectiveness of care as in (1) and the appropriateness of interventions to meet individual needs.

(6) The unit-based nurse will identify the need to refer the patient to other members of the multidisciplinary team, will act where necessary as a co-ordinator of the multi-disciplinary team, and will communicate appropriate information.

(7) The unit-based nurse will facilitate continuity of care following discharge/transfer consulting with the community liaison nurse where indicated.

NURSING

(8) The unit-based nurse documents accurately all aspects of professional practice.

5. OUTCOMES

(1) The patient and family report that post-operative pain was effectively controlled in accordance with the patient's individual needs. They will also feel that their needs for education and for practical and emotional support were met.

(2) The nurse reports that he or she had access to resources as listed and was able to follow the described professional practice. The nurse also considers that he or she was able to meet the needs of the patient and family by providing individualized pain control to relieve post-operative pain, and by offering information and support.

(3) The documentation system will show evidence that resources were used and professional practice was followed to provide individualized and effective post-operative pain control. There will be evidence that the patient and family's needs for education and for practical and emotional support were met.

REFERENCES

Bonica, J. (1980) *Cancer Pain*. Raven Press, New York.

Cohen, F. L. (1980) Postsurgical pain relief: patients' status and nurses' medication choices. *Pain*, **9**, 265–74.

Cartwright, P. D. (1985) Pain control after surgery: a survey of current practice. *Annals of the Royal College of Surgeons of England*, **67**, 13–16

Liebeskind, J. C. & Melzack, R. (1987) The International Pain Foundation: Meeting on the need for education in pain management. *Pain*, **30**, 1–2.

McCaffrey, M. (1979) *Nursing Management of the Patient with Pain*. J.B. Lippincott, Philadelphia.

Royal College of Surgeons & College of Anaesthetists (1990) *Report of the Working Party On Pain after Surgery*. Royal College of Surgeons of England/College of Anaesthetists, London.

CARE OF PATIENTS WITH A SURGICAL WOUND

1. STANDARD STATEMENT

Patients who have surgical wounds will receive comprehensive assessment and appropriate nursing interventions to minimize complications and to promote wound healing and comfort.

2. RATIONALE

Surgery is a major form of treatment for cancer, initially as a potentially curative procedure and subsequently as a debulking or palliative procedure. A wound can be described as an injury made by a cut or blow to tissue including piercing the skin and a surgical wound is one which has been performed in a controlled fashion in order to repair or rectify diseased or damaged tissue.

Patients undergoing surgery have a variety of needs as a result of the cancer diagnosis and concerns about potentially deforming surgery. Therefore, facilitating an uncomplicated post-operative recovery is doubly important both from a physiological viewpoint and in order to promote patients' psychological well-being and confidence in treatment. Wound management, therefore, requires a multidisciplinary approach involving the nurse, pharmacist, dietitian, doctor, physiotherapist and infection control nurse (Johnson, 1988). Nurses play a key role in promoting patient comfort and symptom control, wound assessment and management, and facilitating optimal conditions for wound healing. Equally important is the role of the nurse in relation to patient and family education about wound care, assessment of the impact of the wound for the patient and enabling the patient to cope with the wound.

3. RESOURCES

(1) The unit-based nurse will have a baseline knowledge of the following:

   (a) The anatomy and physiology of the skin and related surgical areas.
   (b) Current research and trends in the management of surgical wounds and wound healing, and their implications for both the patient and family and related nursing care.
   (c) The principles of asepsis and infection control.
   (d) Factors influencing wound healing, including nutrition, drug therapies (e.g. steroids), previous radiotherapy, other illnesses (e.g. diabetes).
   (e) The various agents and dressings available for the management of surgical wounds and their appropriate, research-based use.
   (f) Wound drainage systems (e.g. Redi-vac, corrugated drains, etc.)
   (g) Methods of skin closure and their implications for nursing care.
   (h) The prevention and control of infection and symptoms of both local and systemic infection.
   (i) Potential complications (e.g. haematoma, seroma, haemorrhage, infection) and their management.

(2) The unit-based nurse will have baseline skills in:

   (a) Communication – to make an assessment of the potential physical effects of surgery and to assist the patient with adaptation to the wound.
   (b) Teaching – to teach the patient and family about wound care, how to change dressings (where appropriate) and the signs and symptoms of infection.

(c) Practical techniques – for example, aseptic dressing technique, accurate observation.

(3) The unit-based nurse will have access to ongoing education and support. The clinical nurse specialist/unit manager will organize supervision, and unit-based teaching sessions, where necessary.

(4) The clinical nurse specialist/unit manager is expected to have detailed knowledge as listed in (1) and skills as in (2). Where the problem has specific management issues/difficulties a clinical nurse specialist/unit manager with specialist knowledge and skills may be identified to act as a consultant for advice and support.

(5) Other members of the multidisciplinary team will be available to act as a source of referral or resource to the patient, family and nurse including the clinical nurse specialist (infection control) dietitian, physiotherapist, pharmacist and members of the patient's medical team.

(6) There will be a range of specialist equipment and therapeutic agents available for the management of surgical wounds including cleansing agents and dressings.

(7) Written information will be available to the patient and family, including booklets on breast surgery, stoma surgery and dietary advice.

(8) Written information will be available to the nurse including *The Royal Marsden Hospital Manual of Clinical Procedures* (Chapter 3, pp. 13–18).

(9) An environment suitable to the needs of the patient will be available, including access to privacy.

(10) An environment to meet the needs/requirements of the nurse (e.g. clean area to prepare dressing trolley etc.) will be provided.

---

4. PROFESSIONAL PRACTICE

(1) The unit-based nurse makes a pre-operative assessment of the following.

   (a) The patient's feelings about the surgery, and his or her expectations of the wound.
   (b) The patient's educational needs regarding the anticipated surgery and resulting wound.
   (c) The endogenous characteristics of the patient which might influence wound healing (e.g. age, other illnesses such as diabetes).
   (d) Other factors which might influence wound healing (e.g. nutritional status, previous radiotherapy, current drug therapies etc.)
   (e) The condition of the patient's skin, particularly in the operative area (e.g. is keloid scarring present? Is there bruising/discoloration?)
   (f) Any allergies (e.g. to plasters, surgical tapes, cleansing agents etc.)

(2) The unit-based nurse makes an initial and ongoing post-operative assessment of the following.

   (a) Signs of haemorrhage and/or haematoma/seroma formation (e.g. bleeding, swelling, pain etc.).
   (b) Signs of infection (e.g. inflammation, pyrexia, odour, discoloured exudate, etc.).

(c) Pain/discomfort associated with the wound.

(d) The adequacy of the blood supply to the wound site and dependent areas.

(e) The position of the wound and any limitations in mobility.

(f) The type of drain(s) used and the amount, colour and consistency of drainage fluid.

(g) The size, depth and stage of healing of the wound (only when it is necessary to change or remove the dressing).

(h) The psychological response of the patient (and family, if appropriate) to the surgery and (where appropriate) to seeing the wound.

(3) The unit-based nurse plans and implements care pre-operatively in conjunction with the patient, family and other members of the multidisciplinary team.

(a) The patient (and family) are offered information concerning pre-operative preparation and what to expect post-operatively (e.g. wound site and dressings, drain(s) etc.)

(b) The patient is prepared for surgery safely, according to unit policy.

(c) The nurse liaises with other members of the multidisciplinary team about referral of patients either as a routine (e.g. physiotherapy and breast surgery patients) or as a result of pre-operative assessment (e.g. dietitian).

(4) The unit-based nurse plans and implements post-operative care in conjunction with the patient, family and other members of the multidisciplinary team.

(a) The wound drainage is monitored and the drain(s) changed or removed as appropriate, according to instructions.

(b) The wound and drain site are observed for signs of local complications and the patient monitored for signs of systemic complications.

(c) Where a complication (e.g. haemorrhage, infection) is suspected or identified the nurse liaises with medical colleagues about the initiation of appropriate treatment.

(d) The wound is aseptically redressed only when necessary using the most appropriate cleansing agent(s) and dressing materials. Where necessary, pressure or supportive bandaging is applied.

(e) The nurse monitors the patient's pain levels and offers analgesia as appropriate.

(f) The adequacy of the sutures is monitored and they are removed after discussion with medical colleagues.

(g) The nurse offers the patient individualized support in order to facilitate adaptation to the wound.

(h) The patient is offered information on what to expect after discharge (e.g. possible swelling, paraesthesia), what to do if complications arise.

(i) The patient is offered information on support services available (e.g. following breast surgery or stoma formation).

(5) The unit-based nurse monitors and evaluates the effectiveness of care as in (1) and the appropriateness of interventions to meet individual needs.

(6) The unit-based nurse will identify the need to refer the patient to other members of the multidisciplinary team where appropriate, will act where necessary as co-ordinator of the multidisciplinary team and will communicate appropriate information.

(7) The unit-based nurse will facilitate continuity of care following discharge/transfer consulting with the community liaison nurse where indicated. Prior to discharge the nurse ensures that the patient and/or family have a contact name and number for follow-up advice and information.

(8) The unit-based nurse documents accurately all aspects of professional practice.

5. OUTCOMES

(1) The patient and family report that the patient's needs relating to the wound were recognized and understood and that his or her needs for education and for emotional and practical support were met.

(2) The nurse considers that he or she had access to the resources as listed and was able to follow the described professional practice. The nurse also reports that the patient's needs relating to the wound were assessed, that complications were minimized and wound healing and comfort promoted.

(3) The documentation system will show evidence that resources were used and professional practice followed to ensure that the patient's needs related to the wound were assessed, that complications were minimized and wound healing and comfort promoted.

REFERENCE

Johnson, A. (1988) Criteria for ideal wound dressings. *Professional Nurse*, **3(6)**, 191–3.

CARE OF PATIENTS WITH A STOMA

1. STANDARD STATEMENT

Patients who have a stoma, either permanent or temporary, will be offered support, information and practical help to enable both themselves (and their families) to care safely and independently for their stoma whilst in the hospital setting and on their return home. Nursing care will be directed towards providing a comprehensive rehabilitation programme to enable patients to integrate wherever possible the management of the stoma into their everyday lives.

2. RATIONALE

A stoma may be formed for a variety of reasons including bowel and bladder cancers, inflammatory bowel disease and fistula formation. There are four main types of stoma: an end loop colostomy (usually permanent), a loop transverse colostomy (usually temporary), an ileal conduit and an ileostomy. The permanency as well as the time for psychological preparation for the surgery varies greatly. Although each individual may need to adjust his or her lifestyle in some way, the approaches they use will differ.

Rehabilitation in cancer care is a process by which individuals are assisted to achieve optimal functioning within the limits imposed by their disease. Nursing care is therefore directed towards providing practical advice and guidance for the day-to-day care of the stoma and, just as importantly, it seeks to facilitate emotional adjustment to an altered body image and the possible changes in daily living. The provision of information and support for both the patient and family is an integral part of assisting the patient to achieve the optimal level of rehabilitation. Nurses need to attempt to give quality of life, instilling confidence in an unhurried atmosphere and encouraging the patient to return to self-respect and independence. Discussing the subject freely creates an understanding and understanding hopefully leads to acceptance (Salter, 1988). With these aims setting precedence, the nurse works within the multidisciplinary team to offer the patient and family a rehabilitation programme enabling them to maintain and/or attain optimal functioning in all dimensions of their lives.

3. RESOURCES

(1) The unit-based nurse will have a baseline knowledge of the following.

   (a) The anatomy and physiology of the gastrointestinal and genito-urinary systems.
   (b) The indications for the formation of a either a permanent or temporary stoma.
   (c) The different types of stoma formed and the physical effects of the formation on the patient.
   (d) The type of surgery performed and the short and long term implications of such surgery (e.g. pain, impotence etc.)
   (e) The psychological impact of the formation of a stoma on a patient.
   (f) The possible effects of the formation of a stoma on the family and family life.
   (g) The possible effects of a stoma on a patient's personal relationships, social activities and work activities.
   (h) The day-to-day management of a stoma — including cleaning the stoma and changing appliances, and the appearance and functioning of a healthy stoma.
   (i) The potential problems associated with a stoma (e.g. herniation, prolapse or retraction of the stoma, excoriation of the parastomal skin).
   (j) The effects of other cancer treatments (e.g. radiotherapy) on a stoma.

NURSING

    (k) Stoma products, their availability and indications for use.
    (l) Current research and its implications for both patient, family and related nursing care.

(2) The unit-based nurse will have baseline skills in:

    (a) Communication – to provide information and support to the patient and family before and after surgery, to use consistent terminology with the patient and family to facilitate understanding and prevent misunderstanding, and to convey a sensitive and empathetic attitude.
    (b) Teaching – to educate the patient and family about the normal structure and function of the gastrointestinal and/or genito-urinary systems and the ways in which this will alter following surgery; to educate the patient and family in the care of the stoma and to supervise the patient during the first stages of managing his or her own stoma.
    (c) Practical techniques – for example, to adapt and handle stoma care products on an individual patient basis and to demonstrate practical techniques to the patient and family.

(3) The unit-based nurse will have access to ongoing education and support. The clinical nurse specialist/unit manager will organize supervision, and unit-based teaching sessions, where necessary.

(4) The clinical nurse specialist (stoma care) will have a detailed knowledge as listed in (1), in particular the current trends and developments in stoma care, the availability of stoma care products and the long term implications of stoma formation for the patient and family. The clinical nurse specialist (stoma care) will also have a wider range of teaching and practical skills, and advanced communication skills in order to assess the initial impact of the proposed surgery on the patient, the patient's suitability for such surgery, and to provide individualized information and support. The clinical nurse specialist will also have skills related to the siting of stomas.

(5) The clinical nurse specialist (stoma care) will be available to act as a resource or source of referral for the patient, family and nurse. He or she will also be available to make an initial assessment of patients who will be undergoing the formation of a stoma and to site the position of the stoma.

(6) Other members of the multidisciplinary team will be available to act as a resource or source of referral to the patient, family and nurse including the appliance department, the stoma care nurse and the medical staff.

(7) There will be a range of equipment available to the patient, family and nurse including a selection of stoma care products, templates, etc.

(8) The nurse will have access to current written information and research concerning the care of a patient with a stoma including the individualized patient teaching plan, *The Royal Marsden Hospital Manual of Clinical Nursing Procedures* (Chapter 37, pp. 423–34).

(9) Written information will be available to the patient and family including information booklets about stomas and stoma care, the ward step-by-step guide to changing the stoma appliance, manufacturers' information leaflets about stoma care, information about support groups outside the hospital (e.g. The British Colostomy Association, The

Urostomy Association, and The Ileostomy Association), and information about the availability of aids and equipment.

(10) An environment suitable to the patient's individual needs will be available (e.g. ensuring privacy).

(11) An environment to meet the requirements of the nurse will be available including access to a single room with a full length mirror.

4. PROFESSIONAL PRACTICE

(1) The clinical nurse specialist (stoma care) makes an initial assessment of the patient. In collaboration with medical colleagues the clinical nurse specialist assesses the patient's suitability for the formation of a stoma. She or he assesses the patient and family's level of knowledge and understanding and provides information and support tailored to their individual needs. After discussion with the medical staff the clinical nurse specialist sites the position of the stoma involving the patient (and family) wherever possible. The patient is followed up by the clinical nurse specialist throughout his or her hospital admission and on discharge.

(2) The unit-based nurse makes an initial and ongoing assessment of the following pre-operatively.

   (a) The patient's and family's knowledge and previous experience of stomas.
   (b) The response of the patient and family to the illness and their understanding of its implications.
   (c) The patient's and family's understanding of the physical, psychological and social implications of the formation of a stoma.
   (d) The patient's and family's needs for information, support and education about both the illness and the proposed surgery.
   (e) The patient's job and work environment, leisure and social activities.
   (f) The patient and family's ability (e.g. their visual acuity and manual dexterity) and willingness to participate in the management and care of the stoma.
   (g) The patient's general physique (e.g. the presence of abdominal folds or large breasts).
   (h) The patient's level of mobility.
   (i) The patient's home environment, the family structure and relationships and the patient's level of emotional support.
   (j) The patient's perceptions of what his or her partner will think/feel about him/her after the surgery, and the presence of, or fears about, sexual difficulties after the surgery.

(3) The unit-based nurse makes an initial and ongoing assessment of the following post-operatively.

   (a) The patient's (and family's) reaction to the stoma (e.g. their interest in the stoma, their willingness to be involved in the care of the stoma, whether the patient feels able to look at the stoma, etc.)
   (b) The physical viability of the stoma (e.g. the appearance of the stoma including its colour, warmth and whether there are signs of local oedema, the position of the stoma and whether it is retracted or prolapsed, the healing and integrity of both the stoma and the parastomal skin, and the nature of the effluent, etc.)

NURSING

(c) The patient's general experience of surgery (e.g. the presence of drains or whether the patient is experiencing pain or nausea).

(4) The unit-based nurse plans and implements pre-operative care in conjunction with the patient, family and other members of the multidisciplinary team.

   (a) The patient and family are given information concerning the physical pre-operative preparation.

   (b) The patient and family are offered general information on what to expect in the post-operative period (e.g. pain, nausea, the presence of drains, nasogastric tubes, the position of the stoma site and the presence of the stoma bag).

   (c) The patient and family are offered information concerning what to expect during their stay in the high dependency unit. The nurse liaises with HDU staff to arrange a pre-operative visit by the unit staff, and if the patient wishes, a visit to the high dependency unit.

   (d) The patient and family are offered specific information related to the surgery (e.g. about changes in the mechanism of elimination).

   (e) The patient and family are offered information, support and an opportunity to discuss the implications of the surgery for the patient's personal life, social and work activities. The nurse liaises with medical colleagues to ensure that the patient's and family's needs are addressed.

   (f) The nurse discusses with the patient and family (where appropriate) the range of thoughts and feelings that they might experience after the surgery, emphasizing that these reactions are normal and can fluctuate in the days, weeks and months following surgery.

   (g) The nurse ensures the patient is physically prepared for surgery liaising with the clinical nurse specialist regarding the siting of the stoma and with the medical staff regarding the bowel preparation.

(5) The unit-based nurse plans and implements post-operative care in conjunction with the patient, family and other members of the multidisciplinary team.

   (a) The nurse observes and assesses the stoma viability.

   (b) Initially, the nurse manages the care of the stoma (e.g. emptying and changing the stoma bags).

   (c) The nurse provides symptomatic relief (e.g. administering analgesia to relieve pain, liaising with medical staff to ensure optimal relief).

   (d) The nurse ensures an adequate nutritional and fluid intake/output (liaising with the dietitian and medical staff as necessary).

   (e) The nurse continues to offer the patient and family information and support tailored to their individual and changing needs.

   (f) The nurse promotes and encourages patient independence and family involvement in care where appropriate (e.g. by encouraging the patient to look at the stoma, by involving the patient in the changing of the stoma bag, etc.)

   (g) The nurse offers specific information regarding the management of the stoma in the patient's home environment including where and how equipment can be disposed of, how and where to obtain appliances and how to obtain exemption certificates.

   (h) Where appropriate the nurse offers the patient information on changes that may need to be made to social, leisure and work activities.

   (i) The patient and family are offered information on the statutory and voluntary services available in the community.

   (j) The nurse ensures wherever possible that the patient has been referred to a stoma care nurse for follow-up in the community.

(6) The unit-based nurse monitors and evaluates the effectiveness of care as in (1) and the appropriateness of interventions to meet individual needs.

(7) The unit-based nurse will identify the need to refer the patient to other members of the multidisciplinary team, will act where necessary as co-ordinator of the multidisciplinary team and will communicate appropriate information.

(8) The unit-based nurse will facilitate continuity of care on discharge/transfer, consulting with the community liaison nurse where indicated, and ensuring that the patient and/or family have a contact name or number for follow-up advice and support.

(9) The unit-based nurse documents accurately all aspects of professional practice.

5. OUTCOMES

(1) The patient and family feel that they were able to care safely and independently for the stoma both in the hospital and on return home. They also feel that their needs for education and for emotional and practical support were met.

(2) The nurse considers that he or she had access to the resources as listed and was able to follow the described professional practice. The nurse also considers that, through the provision of education, information and support he or she was able to meet the needs of the patient and family enabling them to care for the stoma safely and independently in hospital and on return home.

(3) The documentation system will show evidence that resources were used and professional practice followed to enable the patient to care safely and independently for the stoma. There will also be evidence that the patient's and family's needs for education and for emotional and practical support were met.

REFERENCES

Salter, M. (1988) (Ed.) *Altered Body Image. The Nurse's Role.* John Wiley, Chichester.

NURSING

PREVENTION OF INFECTION FOR IMMUNOCOMPROMISED PATIENTS

1. STANDARD STATEMENT

Nursing care of the immunocompromised patient is directed towards minimizing the development of hospital-acquired infection and minimizing the risk of auto infection. Patients who develop an infection will receive prompt and appropriate treatment. The patient and family will be offered comprehensive information and support.

2. RATIONALE

The human body is challenged daily by potentially pathogenic organisms. Yet the majority of the population, those who are immunocompetent, for the most part continue to function unaffected. Cancer and its treatments have tremendous implications for the immune system; specifically treatments such as certain radiotherapy and chemotherapy regimes can cause immunosuppression to the extent that those same organisms may lead to potentially life threatening infection (Kelly, 1983). Thus the prevention and prompt treatment of any infection in an immunocompromised host is of primary importance.

Infections may arise from either exogenous (acquired) or endogenous (auto) sources. Nursing care encompasses both aspects. In the first instance, interventions aim to decrease exposure to pathogens. Nurses are in an excellent position to teach patients ways in which they may decrease their chance of infection; this can be tailored towards the individual's learning style, priorities, wishes and capabilities. With regard to auto infection, the nurse utilizes the above educational approach as well as astute observational skills. Without intact immunological responses, many of the usual signs and symptoms of infection are veiled and alternative assessment may be required. If infection is identified, the nurse notifies the attending physician and facilitates prompt treatment. Because of the seriousness of the complication, the nurse utilizes crisis intervention skills in supporting not only the patient, but also the family. Although infection is a physiological phenomenon, its impact is all encompassing, requiring a holistic multidisciplinary approach.

3. RESOURCES

(1) The unit-based nurse will have a baseline knowledge of the following.

   (a) The causes of acquired and auto infection as they relate to the immuno-compromised patient.
   (b) The methods of preventing such infections.
   (c) The assessment of infection in order to facilitate early detection.
   (d) The action to be taken both routinely and in an emergency situation such as that of septic shock, cardiac or respiratory arrest.
   (e) The commonly used anti-bacterial, anti-viral and anti-fungal therapies and their side-effects.
   (f) The policies and procedures as relate to the control of infection, for example as in *The Royal Marsden Hospital Manual of Clinical Nursing Procedures* (Chapter 3, pp. 13–18, Chapter 4, pp. 19–70).
   (g) The possible impact of this problem on the psychological wellbeing and social relationships of the patient and family, particularly the effects of isolation and limited contact.

(2) The unit-based nurse will have baseline skills in:

    (a) Communication – for effective communication with the patient, family and other health professionals to ensure that all possible measures are taken to prevent or treat infection.

    (b) Teaching – for effective education of the patient and family as to the causes of infection, the methods of preventing infection and recognition of early signs of infection.

    (c) Practical techniques – in preventing infection (e.g. effective reverse barrier nursing technique), in observing for early signs of infection (e.g. observation of the buccal mucosa), in screening for infection (e.g. taking swabs, blood specimens) and practical skills in the administration of pharmacological therapies.

(3) The unit-based nurse will have access to ongoing education and support. The clinical nurse specialist/unit manager will organize supervision, and unit-based teaching sessions, where necessary.

(4) The clinical nurse specialist/unit manager is expected to have a detailed knowledge as listed in (1) and skills as in (2). Where the problem has specific management issues or difficulties, or has become persistent and intractable, a clinical nurse specialist/unit manager with specialist knowledge and skills may be identified to act as a consultant for advice and support.

(5) The patient, family and nurse will have access to a member of their medical team to discuss issues related to the prevention and treatment of infection. This medical team member will prescribe pharmacological therapies.

(6) The clinical nurse specialist (infection control) and the Infection Control Officer will be available to act as a resource and source of referral for the patient, family and nurse.

(7) Other members of the multidisciplinary team (e.g. the domestic manager and the CSSD manager) will be available to act as a resource.

(8) There will be a range of equipment available for the prevention and detection of infection (e.g. hand washing facilities, protective clothing, swabs, blood bottles etc.)

(9) There will be a range of commonly used pharmacological substances/therapies for the control and treatment of infection.

(10) The unit-based nurse will have access to the written policies and procedures as they relate to infection control.

(11) There will be written information about infection control available for the patient and family – for example, a leaflet about the management of Hickman lines, and booklets about chemotherapy and radiotherapy.

(12) Patients will have to access to clean shower, bath and toilet facilities, and to a clean ward environment.

(13) The nurse will have access to a clean ward environment including hand washing facilities.

NURSING

4. PROFESSIONAL PRACTICE

(1) The unit-based nurse makes an initial and ongoing assessment of the following.

   (a) Relevant history of previous infections and pharmacological history.
   (b) Current presence and site of infection.
   (c) Current pharmacological therapy or therapies (if any).
   (d) Vital signs (according to hospital policy).
   (e) The patient's own description of physical condition which might indicate early infection.
   (f) The patient and family's understanding of the control of infection and desire to become involved in care planning and implementation. The patient's own preferences should be taken into account (wherever appropriate) when planning care.
   (g) The actual and potential impact of this problem on the psychological wellbeing and social relationships of the patient and family.

(2) The unit-based nurse plans and implements care in conjunction with the patient, family and other members of the multidisciplinary team.

   (a) The nurse attempts to prevent infection through maintaining a pathogen reduced environment (by following hospital policy) and by offering education and support to the patient and family.
   (b) The nurse attempts to detect infection through regular assessment, as (1), and teaching the patient self-examination to identify early signs of infection.
   (c) When a potential infection is suspected, the nurse informs the relevant clinician.
   (d) When an infection is suspected and/or positively identified the nurse implements the appropriate pharmacological or non-pharmacological therapies, in conjunction with the medical staff and other members of the multidisciplinary team, to treat the infection and provide symptomatic relief.
   (e) The nurse, in collaboration with medical colleagues, ensures that early signs of potential toxicity due to the pharmacological treatment of infection (e.g. renal failure, ototoxicity) are identified and acted upon immediately.
   (f) The nurse, in collaboration with medical colleagues, ensures the early recognition and prompt appropriate treatment of complications which can result from severe infection (e.g. septicaemic shock, respiratory or cardiac arrest) or from the pharmacological treatment of infection (i.e. drug toxicity).
   (g) When planning for the patient's discharge the nurse assesses the patient's and family's understanding of the need to continue to protect the patient from infection and to check for signs of early infection.

(3) The unit-based nurse monitors and evaluates the effectiveness of care as in (1) and the appropriateness of interventions to meet individual needs.

(4) The unit-based nurse will identify the need to refer the patient to other members of the multidisciplinary team, will act where necessary as a co-ordinator of the multidisciplinary team, and will communicate appropriate information.

(5) The unit-based nurse will facilitate continuity of care following discharge/transfer consulting with the community liaison nurse where indicated.

(6) The unit-based nurse documents accurately all aspects of professional practice.

5. OUTCOMES

(1) The patient and family report that all possible precautions were taken to reduce the risk of infection, but where the patient did become infected they feel that appropriate treatment was implemented promptly. The patient and family feel that their information and support needs were met.

(2) The nurse considers that he or she had access to the resources as listed and was able to follow the described professional practice. The nurse also considers that hospital-acquired infection was prevented and that the incidence of auto infection was kept to a minimum. The nurse reports that infected patients received prompt and appropriate treatment and that the information and support needs of the patient and family were met.

(3) The documentation system will show evidence that resources were used and professional practice followed to prevent the occurrence of hospital-acquired infection and to minimize the incidence of auto infection. There will be evidence that infected patients received prompt and appropriate treatment and the information and support needs of the patient and family were met.

(4) The incidence of detected infection on each unit will be below the national infection rate.

REFERENCE

Kelly, J. O. (1983) Neutropenia and thrombocytopenia. *Cancer Nursing*, **6(6)**, 487–94.

NURSING REHABILITATION CARE

1. STANDARD STATEMENT

The nursing care of patients attending the rehabilitation unit is directed towards meeting the physical, psychological, spiritual, social, educational and vocational needs of patients. Individualized and family-centred programmes are used to enable individuals to achieve their maximum potential within the limits imposed by their disease and/or its treatment.

2. RATIONALE

Every human being, no matter how sick, has a finite life expectancy and there is something that can be done to improve quality of remaining life. For rehabilitation to be effective or meaningful it must deal with the essential qualities that are not definable in physical terms (Gunn, 1984). Realistic hope is an essential element in the lives of those with cancer. By providing emotional support, understanding and patient teaching about the disease and treatment, oncology nurses may enhance hope and the desire for living with and among patients and their families (Hickey, 1986).

The role of the nurse in cancer prevention includes assessment, teaching, counselling, discharge planning and co-operation (Ahana & Takeuchi, 1978). However the focus of cancer nursing should be broadened beyond the prevention, early detection and treatment of cancer to include the practice and outcomes of rehabilitation in the care of the individual with cancer (Mayer & O'Connor, 1989). Rehabilitation is not just the responsibility of the nurse. It is imperative that the skills of the multidisciplinary team are utilized in the provision of co-ordinated care. It is however, the responsibility of the nurse to be aware of the various supportive measures available and to refer to the appropriate discipline.

3. RESOURCES

(1) The unit-based nurse will have a baseline knowledge of the following.

  (a) The principles of rehabilitation.
  (b) Cancer and its treatment.
  (c) The physical, psychological and social implications of cancer for a patient and his or her family.
  (d) Patient education.
  (e) The role of other members of the multidisciplinary team in rehabilitation.
  (f) The principles of effective team-work.
  (g) Symptom control, wound care and the management of chronic oedema.
  (h) The principles of holistic care.
  (i) Supportive therapies.
  (j) Family-centred care.
  (k) Sociology and psychology as related to health care.
  (l) The voluntary and statuary resources available in the community for the patient and his or her family.

(2) The unit-based nurse will have baseline skills in:

  (a) Communication – for effective communication with the patient and family to ensure accurate assessment of the their needs and to relieve anxiety and distress, and also for effective communication with other health care professionals and agencies.

(b) Teaching – in order to educate and demonstrate care to patients, families and other staff.

(c) Practical techniques – in order to meet the varying needs of patients and their families.

(3) The unit-based nurse will have access to ongoing education and support. The clinical nurse specialist/unit manager will organize supervision, and unit-based teaching sessions, where necessary.

(4) The clinical nurse specialist (rehabilitation) will have detailed knowledge and skills as listed in (1) and (2) and will be available to act as a resource or source of referral within the unit and throughout the hospital.

(5) Other members of the multidisciplinary team will be available to act as a resource or source of referral to the patient, family and nurse.

(6) There will be a range of equipment available to the patient, family and nurse.

(7) The nurse will have access to current written information and research related to rehabilitation.

(8) Written information will be available to the patient and family, including the rehabilitation services leaflet and patient information booklets.

(9) An environment suitable to the patient's individual needs will be available (e.g. giving access to privacy and a non-clinical setting including single rooms for patients, kitchen and a room for supportive therapies).

4. PROFESSIONAL PRACTICE

(1) The unit-based nurse in conjunction with other members of the multidisciplinary team makes an initial and ongoing assessment of the following.

(a) The patient's disease status and any current or past treatments.

(b) The patient's physical, psychological, spiritual, social, educational and vocational needs.

(c) The patient's understanding of the disease and its prognosis, and perception of his or her needs.

(d) The family's understanding of the patient's disease and its prognosis, and the family's needs for information, education and support.

(e) The patient's home environment, the family structure and relationships and the support systems available in the home.

(f) The patient's and family's past and present coping strategies.

(g) The patient's and family's work, social and leisure activities.

(h) The patient's past achievements and future aspirations.

(i) The patient's social interaction within the unit environment and with other patients.

(j) The patient's and family's needs related to discharge (e.g. community services, support groups).

(2) The unit-based nurse analyses the assessment and prioritizes care in conjunction with the patient, family and other members of the multidisciplinary team.

(3) The unit-based nurse plans and implements care in conjunction with the patient, family and other members of the multidisciplinary team by:

(a) Fostering a caring environment where holistic care is stimulated.

(b) Ensuring that the patient receives positive feedback in order to promote self esteem.

(c) Encouraging and motivating the patient in order to establish a positive attitude towards self-care.

(d) Encouraging and promoting self-care through the provision of education that is adapted to the individual capabilities of each patient.

(e) Assisting the patient where appropriate to adapt or adjust to the limitations imposed by cancer and/or its treatment.

(f) When the patient is unable to meet his or her own physical needs, assisting the patient to fulfil these as appropriate.

(g) Encouraging the patient to utilize previous coping strategies and to develop new strategies as necessary.

(h) Acting as patient advocate and mediating between patient and family where appropriate.

(i) Encouraging the patient to plan his or her own daily routine in line with goals set by the multidisciplinary team where appropriate.

(j) Promoting patient and family involvement in supportive therapies.

(k) Co-ordinating recreational activities on the unit.

(l) Offering the patient and family information and support tailored to their individual and changing needs.

(3) The unit-based nurse monitors and evaluates the effectiveness of care as in (1) and the appropriateness of interventions to meet individual needs.

(4) The unit-based nurse will identify the need to refer the patient to other members of the multidisciplinary team, will attend multidisciplinary team meetings and case conferences, will act as co-ordinator where appropriate and will communicate necessary information.

(5) The unit-based nurse facilitates continuity of care on discharge/transfer consulting with other members of the multidisciplinary team and the community liaison nurse where indicated, and ensuring that the patient and family have a contact name and/or number for follow-up advice and support.

(6) The unit-based nurse documents accurately all aspects of professional practice.

5. OUTCOMES

(1) The patient and family report that the patient achieved his or her maximum potential within the limits imposed by cancer. They also report that their needs for education and for practical and emotional support were met.

(2) The nurse reports that he or she had access to the resources as listed and was able to follow the described professional practice. The nurse also considers that, through individualized and family-centred programmes, the patient achieved his or her maximum potential within the limits imposed by cancer.

(3) The documentation system will show that resources were used and professional practice followed in order that, through individualized and family-centred programmes, the patient achieved his or her maximum potential within the limits imposed by cancer.

REFERENCES

Ahana, D. & Takeuchi, A. (1978) Rehabilitation in cancer: concepts and applications. In *Dynamics of Oncology Nursing*, (Ed. by P. Durkenhalter & D. Donley), pp. 174–207. McGraw-Hill, New York.

Gunn, A. (1984) *Cancer Rehabilitation*, Raven Press, New York.

Hickey, S. (1986) Enabling hope. *Cancer Nursing*, **9**, 133–7.

Mayer, D. & O'Connor, L. (1989) Rehabilitation of persons with cancer: an ONS statement. *Oncology Nursing Forum*, **16(3)**, 433.

Standards of Care

Occupational Therapy

GENERAL STANDARD FOR OCCUPATIONAL THERAPY

1. STANDARD STATEMENT

Occupational therapy is directed towards enabling patients to achieve and maintain their optimum level of independence in all areas of their daily lives.

2. RATIONALE

Cancer can cause disability and dysfunction in all areas of a person's life – physical, functional, psychological and social (Strong, 1987). In many cases, a person's functional ability will be affected by the primary tumour as well as by metastases and the treatment he or she is currently receiving, or has had in the past. Mehls (1983) points out that 'the patient with cancer is often overwhelmed by the global effects of the disease on himself and his family'. Occupational therapy can be instrumental in re-establishing a person's self-confidence and independence by helping him/her to identify attainable short term and long term goals, and working towards achieving these.

3. RESOURCES

(1) A State Registered occupational therapist is available to give advice, information and/or treatment.

(2) The occupational therapist will have a background knowledge of oncology and the effects of the disease and treatment on the functional ability of the patient. The occupational therapist will also have a knowledge of the principles of occupational therapy intervention and the resources available to the patient and family in the community.

(3) The occupational therapist will have skills in:

(a) Communication – for effective liaison with other members of the multidisciplinary team, for accurate identification of priorities of treatment and to plan treatment with patients.
(b) Teaching – to teach patients and families about wheelchair mobility and handling, to teach relaxation techniques and to participate in clinical unit teaching programmes.
(c) Practical techniques – for the safe use of equipment and for splinting, etc.

(4) A referral system will be in operation.

(5) The occupational therapist will have access to ongoing education programmes and support to ensure maintenance of the knowledge and skill base and to facilitate updated practice. The Group Head Occupational Therapist will organize departmental teaching sessions as appropriate.

(6) Other members of the multidisciplinary team will be available to act as a resource and source of referral to the patient, family and occupational therapist including the medical staff, community occupational therapist, physiotherapist, etc.

(7) The occupational therapist will have access to, and the co-operation of, the catering department for the provision of appropriate foodstuffs for patient assessment.

(8) A range of 'Standards of Care' for specialist areas of occupational practice will be available to occupational therapy staff.

(9) The occupational therapist will have access to medical information about all patients with occupational therapy needs.

(10) The occupational therapist will have access to a range of standardized aids and adapted equipment for assessment and treatment purposes.

(11) The occupational therapist will have written information available to the patient and family including relevant instructions and safety precautions for any equipment loaned and written advice on how to cope with specific problems (e.g. dressing techniques for patients with hemiplegia).

(12) Written information will be available to the occupational therapist, for example the British Association of Occupational Therapists (BAOT) guidelines for home assessment.

(13) The occupational therapist will have access to secretarial support.

(14) The occupational therapy department will have access to an area that includes:

- a kitchen
- a bathroom and toilet
- a bedroom
- a general treatment area
- storage facilities
- office accommodation and office equipment including a telephone.

(15) The occupational therapist will have available a documentation system to record professional practice. This record will be in the POMR (Problem Orientated Medical Record) format.

4. PROFESSIONAL PRACTICE

(1) Upon referral the occupational therapist makes an initial and ongoing assessment of the following.

(a) Physical status including muscle strength, joint range, muscle tone, sensation, and pain.

(b) Functional status including level of self-care, mobility, perceptual abilities, work or school activities, and leisure and recreational activities.

(c) Psychological status including insight into illness and prognosis, motivation for rehabilitation and cognitive abilities.

(d) Social status including home situation, availability of support systems, and the carer's insight and ability.

(2) The occupational therapist analyses the assessment and offers advice and/or agrees to a plan of treatment with the patient and family.

(3) The occupational therapist implements a plan of treatment based on the needs identified in the assessment.

(4) The occupational therapist co-ordinates such interventions with other members of the multidisciplinary team including medical staff, nursing staff and physiotherapists to ensure that the optimum level of function is attained and maintained.

(5) The occupational therapist evaluates the effectiveness of treatment by reassessing the patient and amends interventions as necessary.

(6) To facilitate continuity of care on discharge, the occupational therapist liaises with the community occupational therapist, the community liaison nurse, the social worker and/or social services, and the general practitioner as appropriate.

(7) The occupational therapist documents all aspects of professional practice in the departmental records and, where appropriate, records occupational therapy treatment or intervention in the medical and/or nursing notes.

5. OUTCOMES

(1) The patient and family consider that the patient has achieved and maintained his or her optimal level of independence. The patient and family feel able to manage independently and safely in the community; they also consider that their needs for information and support were met.

(2) The occupational therapist considers that he or she had access to the resources as listed and was able to follow the described professional practice. The occupational therapist also considers that the patient achieved his or her optimum level of independence and that the patient and family were able to manage independently and safely in the community.

(3) The documentation shows evidence that the patient achieved and maintained his or her optimal level of independence. There will also be evidence that the patient and family felt able to manage independently and safely in the community and that their needs for information and support were met.

REFERENCES

Mehls, J. D. (1983) Occupational therapy as a component of cancer rehabilitation. In *Progress in Cancer Control III : A Regional Approach*, Alan Liss Inc., New York.

Strong, J. (1987) Occupational therapy and cancer rehabilitation. *British Journal of Occupational Therapy*, **50(1)**, 4–6.

STANDARD FOR PATIENTS UNDERGOING TREATMENT FOR BRAIN TUMOURS

1. STANDARD STATEMENT

Occupational therapy for patients undergoing treatment for brain tumours is directed towards improving and/or maintaining independence and productivity in all areas of life.

2. RATIONALE

The presentation of a patient with a brain tumour can vary greatly, depending on the character, rate of growth and site of the neoplasm. Problems which will lead to impairment of a person's ability to cope independently include hemiplegia, sensory deficits, impaired balance and co-ordination, and perceptual and cognitive difficulties (Walton, 1989).

Mehls (1983) points out that 'the patient with cancer is often overwhelmed by the global effects of the disease on himself and his family'. Occupational therapy can be instrumental in re-establishing a person's self-confidence. It can also help to improve and/or maintain independence and productivity in all areas of life by helping the patient to identify attainable short term and long term goals, which they can work towards achieving.

3. RESOURCES

(1) A State Registered occupational therapist is available to give advice, information and/or treatment.

(2) The occupational therapist will have a knowledge of the pathology of brain tumours and the medical treatment methods employed by the hospital and the potential side-effects of these. The occupational therapist will also have a knowledge of the principles of occupational therapy intervention in neurological disorders and the resources available to the patient and family in the community.

(3) The occupational therapist will understand the treatment régimes of the occupational therapy department for the management of patients being treated for brain tumours.

(4) The occupational therapist will have skills in:

   (a) Communication – for effective liaison with other members of the multidisciplinary team and community services and to involve the patient's family or other carers.
   (b) Teaching – to teach patients and families about wheelchair mobility and handling, and to teach dressing techniques for the hemiplegic person.
   (c) Practical techniques – for the safe use of equipment and for splinting, etc.

(5) A referral system will be in operation.

(6) The occupational therapist will have access to ongoing education programmes and support to ensure maintenance of the knowledge and skill base and to facilitate updated practice. The Group Head Occupational Therapist will organize departmental teaching sessions as appropriate.

(7) Other members of the multidisciplinary team will be available to act as a resource and source of referral to the patient, family and occupational therapist including the medical staff, community occupational therapist, physiotherapist, etc.

(8) Wherever possible a system for liaison with outpatient department clinics will be available.

(9) The occupational therapist will have access to and the co-operation of the catering department for the provision of appropriate foodstuffs for patient assessment.

(10) A range of 'Standards of Care' for specialist areas of occupational practice will be available to occupational therapy staff.

(11) Occupational therapists will have access to medical information about all patients with occupational therapy needs.

(12) The occupational therapist will have access to a range of standardized aids with a variable height plinth and assessment equipment, for example COTNAB (Chessington Occupational Therapy Neurological Assessment Battery).

(13) The occupational therapist will have written information available to the patient and family including relevant instructions and safety precautions for any equipment loaned and written advice on how to cope with specific problems (e.g. dressing techniques for patients with hemiplegia).

(14) The occupational therapist will have access to specialized neurological assessment forms.

(15) Written information will be available to the occupational therapist – for example the British Association of Occupational Therapists (BAOT) guidelines for home assessment.

(16) The occupational therapist will have access to secretarial support.

(17) The occupational therapy department will have access to an area that includes:

- a kitchen
- a bathroom and toilet
- a bedroom
- a general treatment area
- storage facilities
- office accommodation and office equipment including a telephone.

(18) The occupational therapist will have available a documentation system to record professional practice. This record will be in the POMR (Problem Orientated Medical Record) format.

4. PROFESSIONAL PRACTICE

(1) The occupational therapist reviews the patient's medical history, known prognosis, intended treatment and whether improvement is anticipated.

(2) The occupational therapist makes an initial and ongoing assessment using a specialized neurological assessment form. The occupational therapist also assesses the patient's activities of daily living and social situation.

(3) If recovery is anticipated, the occupational therapist makes a further specialized assessment – for example, COTNAB which looks particularly at upper limb function, perceptual difficulties and the patient's ability to perform a task and follow instructions.

(4) The occupational therapist analyses the assessment and agrees a to plan of treatment with the patient and family. Treatment may be necessary for any of the following problems.

    (a) **Hemiplegia** – treatment is directed towards:

- counteracting neglect of the hemiplegic side by orientation to that side
- improving asymmetry and poor balance by weight transfer and training for balance
- facilitation of normal movement patterns by inhibition of spasticity and avoidance of associated reactions
- facilitation of selective hand and arm function and inhibiting mass movements
- encouraging co-ordination of both hands through bilateral activities.

    (b) **Sensation difficulties** – when recovery is anticipated, the occupational therapist uses activities to promote function, for example, use of different textures or bilateral activities. The occupational therapist also offers the family advice and education on measures to ensure safety.

    (c) **Steroid-induced myopathy** – when patients experience permanent muscle weakness the occupational therapist provides aids such as a raised toilet seat or bath hoist as appropriate in order to promote independence.

    (d) **Balance and co-ordination difficulties** – the occupational therapist grades activities according to the patient's ability and potential for recovery – for example, working from a large to a small base of support, and encouraging rhythmical movements. The occupational therapist also offers instruction on relaxation techniques as tension and frustration can worsen the problems.

    (e) **Perceptual problems** – the approach used in the treatment of perceptual problems again depends on the prognosis. Where recovery is anticipated, activities requiring practice of perceptual problems are used. Where palliative care is more appropriate, the occupational therapist takes a generally functional approach treating the symptom rather than the cause, teaching the patient repetitive practice of a particular task usually a self-care activity. The occupational therapist also ensures that the family and other health care professionals are aware of both the problem and its management.

    (f) **Cognitive problems** – when patients experience cognitive deficits such as concentration difficulties and memory loss the occupational therapist initiates activities modelled on parts of the COTNAB assessment, pen and paper exercises and memory games. Where a patient is hoping to return to work, activities are incorporated that simulate the working environment.

(6) If the patient's condition deteriorates due to tumour progression, after discussion with the patient, family, medical staff and other appropriate members of the multidisciplinary team, the emphasis of occupational therapy intervention is changed and directed towards palliative care.

(7) The occupational therapist co-ordinates such interventions with other members of the multidisciplinary team including medical staff, nursing staff and physiotherapists to ensure that the optimum level of function is attained and maintained.

(8) The occupational therapist evaluates the effectiveness of treatment by continually reassessing the patient and amends interventions as necessary.

(9) In order to facilitate continuity of care on discharge, the occupational therapist liaises with the community occupational therapist, the community liaison nurse, the social worker and/or social services, and the general practitioner as appropriate. The

OCCUPATIONAL THERAPY

occupational therapist carries out a home assessment with the patient prior to discharge if this is appropriate.

(10) The occupational therapist documents all aspects of professional practice in the departmental records and where appropriate records occupational therapy treatment or intervention in the medical and/or nursing notes.

5. OUTCOMES

(1) The patient and family consider that the patient has improved and/or maintained independence and productivity in all areas of life. The patient and family feel that their needs for information and support were met.

(2) The occupational therapist considers that he or she had access to the resources as listed and was able to follow the described professional practice. The occupational therapist also considers that the patient improved and/or maintained independence and productivity in all areas of life, and that the patient's and family's needs for information and support were met.

(3) The documentation shows evidence that the patient improved and/or maintained independence and productivity in all areas of life. There will also be evidence that the patient and family's needs for information and support were met.

(4) Where the patient's medical condition deteriorates, there will be evidence that appropriate palliative measures were taken.

REFERENCES

Mehls, J. D. (1983) Occupational therapy as a component of cancer rehabilitation. In *Progress in Cancer Control III: A Regional Approach*, Alan Liss, New York.

Walton, Lord (1989) *Essentials of Neurology*, 6th edn. Churchill Livingstone, London.

STANDARD FOR PATIENTS WITH BREAST CANCER

1. STANDARD STATEMENT

Occupational Therapy for patients diagnosed with breast cancer is directed towards enabling patients to achieve and maintain their optimum level of independence in all areas of their daily lives.

2. RATIONALE

A person who has been diagnosed with breast cancer may undergo a variety of treatment régimes. The functional ability and range of movement of the affected arm and shoulder has the potential to be altered by extensive surgery, breast reconstruction and radiotherapy. Those who face metastatic or recurrent breast disease may also experience wider range of functional difficulties as a result of the disease process and palliative treatment regimes. Dietz (1981) points out that such individuals 'must be helped to maintain, in accordance with their potential, maximum independence in physical function or work performance'.

Occupational therapy can be instrumental in improving and/or maintaining independence in all areas of daily living by helping the individual, with early or metastatic breast disease to identify long and short term goals and to work towards these.

3. RESOURCES

(1) A State Registered occupational therapist is available to give advice, information and/or treatment.

(2) The occupational therapist will have a knowledge of the anatomy and physiology of the breast and shoulder joint, and of the implications of breast cancer treatment and advanced disease on a patient's functional ability. The occupational therapist will also have a knowledge of the principles of occupational therapy intervention and the resources available to the patient and family in the community.

(3) The occupational therapist will have skills in:

    (a) Communication – for effective liaison with other members of the multidisciplinary team, for accurate identification of priorities of treatment and to plan treatment with patients.

    (b) Teaching – to teach the patient and family relaxation techniques and to demonstrate dressing techniques to patients with lymphoedema.

    (c) Practical techniques – for example, for the handling and correct use of equipment and wheelchairs.

(4) A referral system will be in operation.

(5) The occupational therapist will have access to ongoing education programmes and support to ensure maintenance of the knowledge and skill base and to facilitate updated practice. The Group Head Occupational Therapist will organize departmental teaching sessions as appropriate.

(6) Other members of the multidisciplinary team will be available to act as a resource and source of referral to the patient, family and occupational therapist including the medical staff, clinical nurse specialists in breast care and lymphoedema, community occupational therapist, physiotherapist, etc.

(7) The occupational therapist will have access to medical information about all patients with occupational therapy needs.

(8) The occupational therapist will have access to a range of standardized aids and adapted equipment for assessment and treatment purposes (e.g. floor mats, tape recorders, etc.).

(9) The occupational therapist will have written information available to the patient and family including, for example, instructions about breathing and relaxation exercises, information related to community services, etc.

(10) The occupational therapist will have access to secretarial support.

(11) An occupational therapy department will be available. This will include:

- a kitchen
- a bathroom and toilet
- a bedroom
- a general treatment area
- storage facilities
- office accommodation and office equipment including a telephone.

(12) The occupational therapist will have available a documentation system to record professional practice. This record will be in the POMR (Problem Oriented Medical Record) format.

4. PROFESSIONAL PRACTICE

(1) Upon referral, the occupational therapist makes an initial and ongoing assessment of the following.

(a) The patient's disease status and previous/current treatments.
(b) The patient's functional status including level of self-care, mobility, work and leisure activities, and domestic activities of daily living.
(c) The patient's physical status including shoulder joint range, pain and the presence of lymphoedema.
(d) The patient's psychological status including insight to illness, motivation and presence of anxiety.
(e) The patient's social status including home situation and environment.

(2) The occupational therapist analyses the assessment and offers advice and/or agrees to a plan of treatment with the patient and family.

(3) The occupational therapist implements a plan of treatment based on the needs identified in the assessment.

(a) The occupational therapist assists the patient to practice activities of daily living and teaches the patient and family alternative strategies/techniques where appropriate.
(b) The occupational therapist offers advice to the patient and family on energy conservation techniques (e.g. spacing activities, rearranging an environment, etc.).
(c) The occupational therapist helps the patient to identify situations where anxiety begins to disrupt normal activities, offers information and/or instruction on a variety

of relaxation strategies/techniques and discusses with the patient and family which methods are the most suited to that individual.

(d) The occupational therapist offers information and education, where appropriate, to the patient and family in the management of wheelchairs and any other equipment required to maintain independence.

(e) The occupational therapist ensures that the family or other carers have adequate support and where necessary arranges support appropriate to their individual needs (e.g. via Social Services or through a cancer support group).

(4) The occupational therapist co-ordinates such interventions with other members of the multidisciplinary team including medical staff, nursing staff and physiotherapists to ensure that the optimum level of function is attained and maintained.

(5) The occupational therapist evaluates the effectiveness of the treatment by reassessing the patient and amends interventions as necessary.

(6) In order to facilitate continuity of care on discharge the occupational therapist liaises with the community occupational therapist, the community liaison nurse, the social worker and/or social services, and the general practitioner as appropriate.

(7) The occupational therapist documents all aspects of professional practice in the departmental records and where appropriate records occupational therapy treatment/intervention in the medical and/or nursing notes.

5. OUTCOMES

(1) The patient and family consider that the patient has achieved and maintained her or his optimal level of independence. The patient and family feel able to manage independently and safely in the community, and they also consider that their needs for information and support were met.

(2) The occupational therapist considers that he or she had access to the resources as listed and was able to follow the described professional practice. The occupational therapist also considers that the patient achieved her or his optimum level of independence and that the patient and family were able to manage independently and safely in the community.

(3) The documentation shows evidence that the patient achieved and maintained her or his optimal level of independence. There will also be evidence that the patient and family felt able to manage independently and safely in the community, and that their needs for information and support were met.

REFERENCES

Dietz, J. H. (1981) *Rehabilitation Oncology*. John Wiley, Toronto.

OCCUPATIONAL THERAPY

Standards of Care

Physiotherapy

GENERAL STANDARD FOR PHYSIOTHERAPY

1. STANDARD STATEMENT

Physiotherapy is directed towards enabling patients to maintain or achieve their maximum potential of functional ability and/or gain symptom control.

2. RESOURCES

(1) A State Registered physiotherapist is available to give advice, information and/or treatment.

(2) Physiotherapists will have access to ongoing education and support. The Group Superintendent Physiotherapist will organize supervision, and department-based teaching sessions where necessary.

(3) A referral system will be in operation, as follows:

   (a) Physiotherapists take both written and verbal referrals from all members of the multidisciplinary health care team.
   (b) Physiotherapists visit every ward every weekday morning (excluding bank and statutory holidays) between 9.00 and 10.30 to receive referrals.
   (c) Referrals can be sent to the physiotherapy department, or phoned in before 5.00 PM. In the case of an urgent referral, a physiotherapist can be bleeped.
   (d) Physiotherapists will attend specialist clinics wherever possible in order to screen for patients with physiotherapy needs, and give advice as appropriate.
   (e) Physiotherapists will attend multidisciplinary ward meetings to collect referrals.
   (f) Physiotherapists will carry bleeps in order that those with specialist skills may receive referrals directly.

   - All non-urgent ward referrals for respiratory physiotherapy will be dealt with within three hours of receipt of the referral. If emergency respiratory referrals are received the physiotherapist will be available to give treatment within one hour, at any time of the day or night. All other referrals received before 3.00 PM will be dealt with on the same day of referral. Referrals received after 3.00 PM may have to wait until the following weekday
   - Referrals for emergency physiotherapy outside 9.00 AM to 5.00 PM, Monday to Friday, must come from physiotherapy or medical staff only. A physiotherapist will

be contactable at any time of the day or night and the referring doctor must speak to the on-call physiotherapist direct.

(4) A referral system to other members of the multidisciplinary team, or other physiotherapy departments, will be in operation.

  (a) Members of the multidisciplinary health care team will take both written and verbal referrals from physiotherapists. These should be documented in the physiotherapy treatment records.

  (b) Referrals to other physiotherapy departments should be in writing, with a copy attached to the physiotherapy treatment record.

(5) A 'feedback' system to the referrer will be operational: verbal or written feedback will be given to the referring health care professional on completion of treatment. A copy of all written reports is attached to the physiotherapy treatment record.

(6) An out-patient appointment system will be in operation.

  (a) Patients referred for out-patient physiotherapy will receive an appointment to see a physiotherapist within one week of receipt of the referral.

  (b) Out-patients may attend for physiotherapy between 9.00 AM and 5.00 PM, Monday to Friday. The timing and frequency of these treatments will be decided by the physiotherapist taking up the referral.

(7) Physiotherapists will have access to medical information about patients with physiotherapy needs.

(8) 'Standards of Care' for specialist areas of physiotherapy practice will be available to physiotherapy staff.

(9) The Chartered Society of Physiotherapy 'Standards of Physiotherapy Practice' will be available to physiotherapy staff.

(10) Physiotherapy advice/information sheets will be available for patients.

(11) A range of aids and equipment is available. A procedure for the loan of equipment is in operation.

(12) A standardized physiotherapy treatment record, which is problem based and recorded in SOAP (Subjective and Objective assessment, Analysis and Plan) format, is used.

(13) The environment available for physiotherapy staff and patients includes the following.

  (a) A designated physiotherapy area accessible to staff and patients.
  (b) Comfortable reception and waiting facilities.
  (c) Private, secure and comfortable treatment areas.
  (d) Facilities for physiotherapy staff (e.g. office areas, changing accommodation, personal lockers).
  (e) Secure storage for physiotherapy treatment records.

  • **NB** The physiotherapy area must comply with the Health and Safety Act, local policies and standards of The Chartered Society of Physiotherapy, whichever is higher.

PHYSIOTHERAPY

---

3. PROFESSIONAL PRACTICE

On receipt of referral the physiotherapist:

(1) Undertakes an initial physiotherapy assessment of the patient, identifying the needs of both the patient and family.

(2) Analyses the assessment and draws up a list of problems relevant to the physiotherapy management.

(3) Agrees with the patient problem orientated goals and related treatment plans.

(4) Implements a plan of physiotherapy management in conjunction with the patient, family and other members of the multidisciplinary team.

(5) Re-assesses the patient throughout the duration of the care episode, re-adjusting the goals and plans according to objective and subjective changes in the patient's condition or circumstances.

(6) Communicates and liaises with other members of the multidisciplinary team and/or other physiotherapy departments to facilitate continuity of care and an optimum level of care.

(7) Documents accurately all elements of the care episode according to the documentation standards of the physiotherapy service.

---

4. OUTCOMES

(1) The patient and family consider that the patient achieved his or her maximum potential of functional ability and/or gained symptom control. They also report that they understood the long term management of any residual disability or dysfunction and that they were satisfied with the care they received.

(2) The physiotherapist considers that he or she had access to the resources as listed and was able to follow the described professional practice. The physiotherapist also reports that the patient achieved his or her maximum potential of functional ability and/or gained symptom control and understood the long term management of any residual disability or dysfunction.

(3) The documentation system will show evidence that resources were used and professional practice followed in order for the patient to achieve maximum potential of functional ability and/or gain symptom control.

STANDARD FOR PATIENTS UNDERGOING BONE MARROW TRANSPLANTATION

1. STANDARD STATEMENT

Physiotherapy for patients undergoing bone marrow transplantation is directed towards minimizing the risk of side-effects and managing these should they occur in order for the patients to regain their maximum potential of functional ability.

2. RATIONALE

Bone marrow transplantation can be part of the treatment protocol for acute leukaemia. It involves treatment with high doses of chemotherapy and/or total body irradiation which completely ablates patients' own bone marrow and therefore the abnormal leukaemic cells. Patients then have either their own or donated bone marrow reinfused. Following bone marrow transplantation patients are nursed in protective isolation until the graft establishes itself (3–6 weeks). During this period the patient may experience several treatment complications including nausea, vomiting, fever, infection, pain and graft versus host disease (GVHD). They also experience a period of profound bone marrow suppression.

The above complications and the psychological and social adjustments of these patients (James, 1987) can lead to a period of inactivity, psychological depression and loss of body protein. Physiotherapy, in the form of prophylactic daily exercise régimes tailored to individual patient needs, is important to maintain the body protein reserves and prevent complications of bed-rest. It also promotes physical and emotional wellbeing (James, 1987) thus enabling patients to regain their maximum functional ability.

3. RESOURCES

(1) A State Registered physiotherapist is available to give advice, information and/or treatment.

(2) The physiotherapist will have knowledge of the physiological effects of and potential problems associated with inactivity and prolonged bed-rest. The physiotherapist will also have an understanding of the potential side-effects associated with high dose chemotherapy, total body irradiation, and related drug therapies.

(3) The physiotherapist will understand the régimes of the physiotherapy department for the management of patients undergoing bone marrow transplantation.

(4) The physiotherapist will have access to ongoing education/support. The Group Superintendent Physiotherapist will organize supervision, and department-based teaching sessions, where necessary.

(5) There will be a referral system to the physiotherapy department for other members of the multidisciplinary team to refer patients before they undergo bone marrow transplantation.

(6) There will be a referral system to other members of the multidisciplinary team, or other physiotherapy departments as follows.

(a) Members of the multidisciplinary health care team will take both written and verbal referrals from physiotherapists. These should be documented in the physiotherapy treatment records.

(b) Referrals to other physiotherapy departments should be in writing, with a copy attached to the physiotherapy treatment record.

(7) There will be a 'feedback' system to the referrer; verbal or written feedback is given to the referring health care professional on completion of treatment. A copy of all written reports is attached to the physiotherapy treatment record.

(8) Physiotherapists will have access to medical information about patients undergoing bone marrow transplantation.

(9) A range of specialist aids and equipment will be available for the management of patients undergoing bone marrow transplantation (e.g. static exercise bicycles in the isolation rooms).

(10) Specific written physiotherapy advice/information will be available to patients undergoing transplantation.

(11) A standardized physiotherapy treatment record, which is problem based and recorded in SOAP (Subjective and Objective assessment, Analysis and Plan) format, will be used.

(12) An environment appropriate to the needs of the patient and the physiotherapist will be available (see page 155, point 13).

(13) The Chartered Society of Physiotherapy 'Standards of Physiotherapy Practice' will be available to physiotherapy staff.

4. PROFESSIONAL PRACTICE

(1) Pre-transplantation, the physiotherapist undertakes an initial assessment including the following.

(a) A review of the patient's medical history including the length and presentation of the illness, any previous oncological treatment and side-effects (particularly any weight loss), the patient's respiratory status and results of recent blood tests.
(b) The patient's home situation (including family support), occupation and leisure activities.
(c) Subjective assessment of the level of activity, physical fitness and wellbeing.
(d) Physical assessment including:

- an exercise tolerance test on a treadmill, to test muscle endurance and the aerobic capacity of the patient
- lung function testing (using a vitalograph) to establish respiratory status.

(2) The physiotherapist analyses the assessment and draws up a list of problems relevant to the physiotherapy management.

(3) The physiotherapist offers advice and/or agrees with the patient problem-orientated goals and related treatment plans.

(4) The physiotherapist implements a plan of physiotherapy treatment in conjunction with the patient and other members of the multidisciplinary team including:

(a) The provision of information about the role of the physiotherapist during all phases of the transplant period, the importance of exercise during this period where normal activity is impossible and the problems associated with bed-rest or inactivity.

(b) Instruction in an exercise régime tailored to the individual's medical condition, ability and preference. This exercise regime is designed to maintain and improve:

- muscle strength
- respiratory and cardiovascular function
- joint range of movement
- body's protein reserves. It is also designed to help with the psychological considerations associated with long term hospitalization.

(5) The physiotherapist reassesses the patient throughout the period of the care episode, readjusting the goals and treatment plans according to the environment (e.g. the protective isolation room) and both objective and subjective changes in the patient's condition. These may include the development of treatment complications such as chest infections, steroidal myopathies, graft versus host disease and nerve palsies.

(6) Prior to discharge from the ward the physiotherapist and patient agree to goals and a treatment plan to maintain progress. This may involve the following.

(a) Continuation of an exercise programme at home by the patient.

(b) Continuation of physiotherapy at the hospital if appropriate and geographically possible.

(c) Referral to a local physiotherapy department for continuation of treatment.

(d) Regular monitoring and re-assessment through out-patient clinics.

(7) The physiotherapist liaises with other members of the multidisciplinary team and/or other physiotherapy departments to facilitate continuity of care and an optimum level of care.

(8) The physiotherapist documents accurately all elements of the care episode according to the documentation standards of the physiotherapy service.

5. OUTCOMES

(1) The patient and family report that the patient achieved maximum functional ability and was able to resume his or her previous work, social and leisure activities. They also report that they understood the need to continue exercise and how to manage any residual dysfunction, and they were satisfied with the care received.

(2) The physiotherapist considers that he or she had access to the resources as listed and was able to follow the described professional practice. The physiotherapist also reports that the patient achieved maximum functional ability and understood the need to continue regular, long term exercise to maintain and further improve functional ability, and how to manage any residual dysfunction.

(3) The documentation system shows evidence that resources were used and professional practice followed in order for the patient to maintain or achieved maximum functional ability. The documentation system also demonstrates side-effects were minimized and managed if they occurred.

PHYSIOTHERAPY

REFERENCE

James, M. C. (1987) Physical therapy for patients after bone marrow transplantation. *Physical Therapy*, **67 (6)**, 946–52.

STANDARD FOR PATIENTS UNDERGOING BREAST SURGERY

1. STANDARD STATEMENT

Physiotherapy for patients who have undergone either surgical dissection of the axillary nodes with or without wide local excision of the breast lump, or mastectomy with or without breast reconstruction is directed towards enabling patients, on discharge from physiotherapy, to continue their exercises and understand the instruction that will enable them, firstly, to regain maximum function ability of the upper limb ipsilateral to the breast surgery and, secondly, to minimize the risk of developing post-operative lymphoedema.

2. RATIONALE

The extent of surgery for breast cancer is dictated by the histology and extent of the disease. Axillary lymph node dissection is frequently employed as either a staging or therapeutic procedure, but is associated with some disability and limitation of function and lymphoedema formation (Kissen *et al.*, 1986). More extensive surgery, such as mastectomy with or without breast reconstruction, may interfere with the pectoralis muscle group and hence also impede function.

A régime of post-operative exercises under the supervision of a physiotherapist, will assist these patients to regain full range of shoulder movement, and improve function sooner (Wingate, 1985). Instruction in the use of the arm post-operatively may facilitate resumption of the patient's usual functional activities, whilst advice on care of the arm given to those at risk of developing lymphoedema may decrease its incidence.

3. RESOURCES

(1) A State Registered physiotherapist is available to give advice, information and/or treatment.

(2) The physiotherapist will have anatomical knowledge of the neck, forequarter, chest wall, breast and lymphatic system; and will understand the surgical procedures commonly used at the hospital and the potential/actual dysfunction arising from these procedures. The physiotherapist will understand the régimes used by the physiotherapy department as they pertain to the breast unit.

(3) Physiotherapists will have access to ongoing education and support. The Group Superintendent physiotherapist will organize supervision and department-based teaching sessions where necessary.

(4) There will be a referral system for other members of the multidisciplinary team to refer patients to the physiotherapist pre-operatively.

(5) There will be a system for the physiotherapist to attend surgical out-patient clinics, and follow-up in-patients at their first post-operative clinic appointment.

(6) There will be a referral system to other members of the multidisciplinary team, or to other physiotherapy departments as follows.

    (a) Members of the multidisciplinary health care team will take both written and verbal referrals from physiotherapists. These should be documented in the physiotherapy treatment records.

PHYSIOTHERAPY

(b) Referrals to other physiotherapy departments should be in writing, with a copy attached to the physiotherapy treatment record.

(7) A 'feedback' system to the referrer; verbal or written feedback is given to the referring health care professional on completion of treatment. A copy of all written reports is attached to the physiotherapy treatment record.

(8) The physiotherapist will have access to medical information about patients undergoing breast surgery.

(9) A range of specialist aids and equipment for the treatment of patients following breast surgery is available.

(10) Specific, written physiotherapy advice/information is available for patients following breast surgery.

(11) A standardized physiotherapy treatment record, which is problem based and recorded in SOAP (Subjective and Objective assessment, Analysis and Plan) format, will be used.

(12) An environment appropriate to the needs of the patient and physiotherapist will be available (see page 155, point 13).

(13) The Chartered Society of Physiotherapy 'Standards of Physiotherapy Practice' will be available to physiotherapy staff.

4. PROFESSIONAL PRACTICE

(1) The physiotherapist gives an explanation to the patient of the importance of physiotherapy following breast surgery, and gains her consent to examination.

(2) The physiotherapist undertakes a pre-operative assessment, which is recorded in the physiotherapy record and includes the following.

(a) A review of relevant past medical history and history of present condition (e.g. previous surgery, radiotherapy and/or chemotherapy).

(b) A subjective assessment of the patient's:

- functional ability
- occupation/work status
- leisure activities
- home situation/family support
- hand dominance.

(c) A physical examination including:

- both the glenohumeral joints, recording the range of movement in the following planes: elevation through flexion; elevation through abduction; medial and lateral rotation.

   NB If bilateral glenohumeral movement in these planes is equal and at full range, a visual estimate of movement is made and recorded. If movement in the glenohumeral joint ipsilateral to the breast disease is restricted the range of movement must be measured with a goniometer, as should all subsequent post-operative measurements.

- The neck, and the chest wall and forequarter ipsilateral to the breast disease, recording abnormalities such as muscle spasm, swelling, decreased range of joint movement and pain.

(3) On the patient's first post-operative day the physiotherapist reiterates the importance of physiotherapy and gains consent to undertake a post-operative assessment of the patient's condition, including the following.

(a) A review of the surgical procedure.
(b) Determination of the patient's level of post-operative pain (by questioning).
(c) A physical examination of:

- the glenohumeral joint ipsilateral to the surgery, recording range of movement through the following planes: elevation through flexion; elevation through abduction; medial and lateral rotation.
- the neck, and the chest wall and forequarter ipsilateral to the surgery recording abnormalities such as swelling, muscle spasm, long thoracic nerve palsy.

(4) The physiotherapist analyses the assessment and draws up a list of problems relevant to the physiotherapy management.

(5) The physiotherapist offers advice and/or agrees with the patient problem orientated goals and related treatment plans.

(6) The physiotherapist implements a plan of treatment in conjunction with the patient, family and other members of the multidisciplinary team. This will include the following.

(a) Teaching the patient to perform regularly progressive standardized shoulder exercises, providing both written and verbal instruction.

NB Set A exercises are commenced on the first post-operative day, Set B exercises when the wound drainage tubes are removed and Set C at the patient's first outpatient clinic appointment, unless complications arise.

(b) While the patient is on the ward, supervising her performing these exercises.
(c) Following axillary dissection, offering verbal and written advice on:

- the prevention of lymphoedema
- who to contact if she notices any lymphoedema.

(d) Offering verbal and written advice on the functional use of the arm.

(7) The physiotherapist reassesses the patient including the following.

(a) Measurement and recording of the glenohumeral joint ipsilateral to the surgery.
(b) Examination of the neck, forequarter and chest wall, and breast and ipsilateral to the surgery, recording:

- any abnormalities such as swelling and muscle spasm
- any post-operative complications such as increased wound drainage, haematoma/seroma formation, wound infection, malposition of breast prosthesis and long thoracic nerve palsy.

(c) Subjective questioning of the patient about her levels of pain.
(d) Review of the patient's medical records and care plans.

(8) The physiotherapist modifies the goals and plan of treatment according to the findings of the continued assessment.

(9) When the patient attends for their first post-operative clinic appointment the patient is assessed by a physiotherapist who will:

   (a) Examine the patient for post operative complications which may affect the function of the shoulder (e.g. seroma, wound infection, cording).
   (b) Measure the range of glenohumeral movement.
   (c) Subjectively assess the patient's level of functional activity.

(10) Depending on the findings of this assessment the physiotherapist agrees new goals and plans with the patient which will enable the patient to regain her maximum functional ability. A further course of physiotherapy is deemed necessary if:

   (a) The patient is to have a course of radiotherapy.
   (b) Pain has increased locally.
   (c) The patient has not regained 75% of her full pre-operative range of movement.
   (d) The patient reports that her level of functional activity is insufficient to allow her to continue activities of daily living at home unaided.

(11) The physiotherapist liaises with other members of the multidisciplinary team and/or other physiotherapy departments to facilitate continuity of care and an optimum level of care.

5. OUTCOMES

(1) The patient and family report that the patient was able to resume her previous work, social and leisure activities. They also report that the patient understood the advice and instruction that would enable her to regain maximum functional ability and minimize the risk of lymphoedema, and were satisfied with the care received.

(2) The physiotherapist considers that he or she had access to the resources as listed and was able to follow the described professional practice. The physiotherapist also reports that the patient understood the advice and instruction that would enable her to regain maximum functional ability and minimize the risk of lymphoedema.

(3) The documentation system will show evidence that resources were used and professional practice followed in order that the patient achieved maximum functional ability of her upper limb, and was given the advice that would minimize the risk of developing lymphoedema.

REFERENCES

Kissen, M. W., Querci della Rovere, G., Easton, D. & Westbury, G. (1986) Risk of lymphoedema following the treatment of breast cancer. *British Journal of Surgery*, **73**, 580–4.

Wingate, L. (1985) Efficiency of physical therapy for patients who have undergone mastectomy. *Physical Therapy*, **65**, 896–900.

STANDARD FOR PATIENTS UNDERGOING PRIMARY RADIOTHERAPY TO THE UPPER AND LOWER EXTREMITIES AND THE HEAD AND NECK REGION

PHYSIOTHERAPY

1. STANDARD STATEMENT

Physiotherapy for patients undergoing primary radiotherapy to the upper and lower extremities or head and neck region is directed towards enabling patients to maintain maximum function both during and following treatment.

2. RATIONALE

Radiotherapy is one of the main medical treatment modalities for cancer. Radiotherapy given to an extremity or the head and neck region will have both short and long term effects upon the tissues within the radiation field. The early effects include an acute skin reaction which may cause pain and skin breakdown. This can lead to limited joint range of movement, poor limb positioning, abnormal gait pattern and decreased functional ability. Physiotherapy management at this stage will help to prevent these short term complications from causing more long term functional disability.

The late effects of radiotherapy include fibrosis of soft tissues and the obliteration of superficial lymphatic and blood vessels. These may lead to limitation of joint range of movement, lymphoedema formation and devascularization of the area (Kissing *et al.*, 1986, Ryttov *et al.*, 1988). Physiotherapy advice and/or intervention may minimize the risk of long term reduction in joint movement and soft tissue extensibility, therefore maintaining optimal function. It may also assist in preventing lymphoedema formation.

3. RESOURCES

(1) A State Registered physiotherapist is available to give advice, information and/or treatment.

(2) The physiotherapist will have anatomical knowledge of the upper and lower extremities and the head and neck region, and an understanding of the potential effects of, and dysfunction arising from, radiotherapy.

(3) The physiotherapist will understand the régimes used by the physiotherapy department for the management of patients receiving radiotherapy.

(4) The physiotherapist will have access to ongoing education and support. The Group Superintendent Physiotherapist will organize supervision and department-based teaching sessions, where necessary.

(5) There will be a referral system for other members of the multidisciplinary team to refer patients at their first radiotherapy planning appointment.

(6) There will be a referral system to other members of the multidisciplinary team, or other physiotherapy departments as follows.

   (a) Members of the multidisciplinary health care team will take both written and verbal referrals from physiotherapists. These should be documented in the physiotherapy treatment records.
   (b) Referrals to other physiotherapy departments should be in writing, with a copy attached to the physiotherapy treatment record.

(7) A 'feedback' system to the referrer; verbal or written feedback is given to the referring health care professional on completion of treatment. A copy of all written reports is attached to the physiotherapy treatment record.

(8) Physiotherapists will have access to medical information about patients undergoing radiotherapy.

(9) A range of specialist aids and equipment is available for patients undergoing radiotherapy.

(10) Specific written physiotherapy advice/information will be available for patients undergoing radiotherapy.

(11) A standardized physiotherapy treatment record, which is problem-based and recorded in SOAP (Subjective and Objective assessment, Analysis and Plan) format, will be used.

(12) An environment appropriate to the needs of the patient and physiotherapist will be available (see page 155, point 13).

(13) The Chartered Society of Physiotherapy 'Standards of Physiotherapy Practice' will be available to physiotherapy staff.

4. PROFESSIONAL PRACTICE

(1) The physiotherapist undertakes an initial assessment including the following.

  (a) A review of the patient's medical history including his or her previous treatment history (i.e. previous surgery, radiotherapy and chemotherapy) and any pre-existing problems in the affected limb, head and neck region.
  (b) Details of radiotherapy are noted including the size of the radiation field, the inclusion of joints within this field and the method of dose fractionation.
  (c) The patient's occupation and leisure activities.
  (d) A subjective assessment of functional ability.
  (e) A physical examination including:

  - active and passive range of movement of all joints of the limb or head and neck region to be irradiated
  - power of muscle groups in the limb or head and neck region to be irradiated
  - gait analysis of patients undergoing radiotherapy to the lower limb
  - possible evidence of lymphoedema in the limb to be irradiated.

(2) The physiotherapist analyses the assessment and draws up a list of problems relevant to the physiotherapy management.

(3) The physiotherapist offers advice and agrees with the patient problem-orientated goals and related treatment plans.

(4) The physiotherapist implements a plan of monitoring, treatment and advice in conjunction with the patient, family and other members of the multidisciplinary team.

(a) Patients undergoing radiotherapy are offered instruction in an exercise régime according to their individual needs. This is designed to maintain normal joint range of movement and muscle power both during and following radiotherapy, hence maintaining functional ability.

(b) The long term effects of radiotherapy are discussed with the patient and the need to continue the exercise régime for at least two years following completion of treatment is emphasized.

(c) The physiotherapist offers advice regarding the potential problem of lymphoedema formation and its prophylaxis.

(5) The physiotherapist reassesses the patient throughout the duration of radiotherapy, re-adjusting the goals and treatment plans according to objective and subjective changes in the patient's condition.

(6) On completion of the course of radiotherapy the physiotherapist and patient agree a plan of physiotherapy to manage any residual dysfunction in the irradiated limb or head and neck region. This may involve:

(a) Continuation of physiotherapy at the hospital if appropriate and geographically possible.

(b) Referral to a local physiotherapy department for continuation of treatment.

(c) Regular assessment when the patient attends for an out-patient clinic appointment and, where necessary, advice and instruction.

(7) The physiotherapist liaises with other members of the multidisciplinary team and/or other physiotherapy departments to facilitate continuity of care and an optimum level of care.

(8) The physiotherapist documents accurately all elements of the care episode according to the documentation standards of the physiotherapy service.

5. OUTCOMES

(1) The patient and family report that the patient maintained his or her maximum potential of functional ability and was able to resume previous work, leisure and social activities. They report that they understood the need for a regular, long term exercise régime and were instructed in the management of potential formation of lymphoedema in the affected limb. The patient and family also report satisfaction with the care received.

(2) The physiotherapist considers that he or she had access to the resources as listed and was able to follow the described professional practice. The physiotherapist also reports that the patient maintained his or her maximum potential of functional ability, understood the need for a regular, long term exercise regime and was instructed in the management of potential formation of lymphoedema in the affected limb.

(3) The documentation system will show evidence that resources were used and professional practice followed in order for the patient to maintain his or her maximum potential of functional ability. There will be evidence that the patient understood the need for a regular, long term exercise régime and was instructed in the management of potential formation of lymphoedema in the affected limb.

PHYSIOTHERAPY

REFERENCES

Kissing, M. W., Querci della Rovere, G., Easton, D. & Westbury, G. (1986) Risk of lymphoedema following the treatment of breast cancer. *British Journal of Surgery*, **73**, 580–4.

Ryttov, N., Holm, N. V., Quist, N. & Buchert-Toft, M. (1988) Influence of adjuvant radiation on the development of late arm lymphoedema and impaired shoulder mobility after masectomy for carcinoma of the breast. *Acta Oncologia*, **27**, 667–70.

Standards of Care

Social Work

ACCESS TO DISABILITY BENEFITS

1. STANDARD STATEMENT

Welfare advice for patients eligible for disability benefits aims to provide information about available resources and practical help to gain access to these.

2. RATIONALE

The average disabled person has a much lower income than the average non-disabled person (Disability Alliance, 1991) According to the Child Poverty Action Group, in 1985 34% of non-pensioner adults with a disability were living in poverty below 50% of average income in comparison with 23% of general population (Oppenheim, 1990). The Family Expenditure Survey (OPCS, 1988/9) found that income from earnings of households with disabled people are low primarily because fewer households with disabled people are working. But where they do work the earnings of all household members, not just the disabled person, are lower than in other households. In addition, it is far more difficult for a disabled person to manage on the same income as someone of the same age who is not disabled. In 1985, the Child Poverty Action Group found that on average adults with a disability were spending an extra £6.10 per week on regular extra costs such as prescriptions, home services, fuel, clothing and bedding (Oppenheim, 1990). Benefits were not always claimed, however, because:

- people do not know about them
- people cannot understand them
- people do not know how to go about claiming them.

The welfare adviser can help patients gain access to appropriate benefits.

3. RESOURCES

(1) The welfare adviser will have knowledge of the following.

    (a) Disability benefits.
    (b) The working procedures of the Department of Social Security (DSS).
    (c) Other specialist agencies.
    (d) Sources of funding.

(2) The welfare adviser will have skills in:

    (a) Communication – to give information and interpret it in a way understandable to the patient.

    (b) Teaching – to educate the patient on benefits and procedures of Department of Social Security in assessing eligibility for benefits, and to educate medical staff on appropriate referrals.

    (c) Practical matters – to follow through benefit applications with patients.

(3) A system for referral and feedback to and from other members of the multidisciplinary team.

(4) The welfare adviser will have access to current technical information on benefits.

(5) Information leaflets for patients and families will be available.

(6) The welfare adviser will have access to a telephone and an appropriate room in order to interview patients in confidence and privacy.

(7) The welfare adviser will have access to professional continuing education.

(8) The welfare adviser will have access to current literature related to disability benefits.

4. PROFESSIONAL PRACTICE

(1) The welfare adviser will undertake the following.

    (a) Making an initial assessment of the benefits for which the patient may be eligible.

    (b) Obtaining a comprehensive assessment of the patient's and family's financial situation – income and outgoings.

    (c) An assessment of the patient's ability to follow any solution to the problem.

(2) The welfare adviser, together with the patient/family, will decide what course of action to take.

    (a) A patient will not be referred without his or her permission.

    (b) The patient will be given the information he or she needs in an understandable way.

    (c) The patient will be helped to understand his or her eligibility for benefits.

    (d) The welfare adviser will mediate between the patient and the benefits agency to minimize potential misunderstandings.

    (e) The welfare adviser will represent the patient's interests and acquire services and benefits that are the patient's right, but which the patient might not be able to negotiate for him or herself.

    (f) The welfare adviser will help the patient through the 'maze' when applying for benefits and negotiate with the DSS.

(3) The welfare adviser will:

    (a) Evaluate interventions and monitor follow-up. Also pursue those initiatives carried out by the patient at specific time periods as discussed with patient.

    (b) Ensure that the patient understands the need for follow-up as above, and will contact the welfare adviser.

    (c) Make case recordings and keep them in a safe place.

5. OUTCOMES

(1) The patient and family report that they were provided with appropriate practical help and information.

(2) The welfare adviser considers that he or she had access to resources required and was able to follow the prescribed professional practice. He or she also reports that the patient and family were provided with practical help and information in order to claim appropriate benefits.

(3) The case records will show evidence that resources were used and professional practice followed to ensure that patients and families were provided with appropriate information, and given appropriate practical help in order to claim the benefits for which they are eligible.

REFERENCES

Disability Alliance (1991) *Disability Rights Handbook*, 16th edn. The Disability Alliance Education and Research Association, London.

Office of Population Censuses and Surveys (OPCS) (1988/9) *Surveys of Disability in Great Britain*, Reports 1–6. HMSO, London.

Oppenheim, C. (1990) *Poverty: The Facts*, Child Poverty Action Group, London.

SOCIAL WORK

FINANCIAL PROBLEMS

1. STANDARD STATEMENT

Welfare advice for patients experiencing financial difficulties aims to provide information about available resources, ways to manage the financial situation, and practical help to minimise financial difficulties.

2. RATIONALE

Financial problems often occur as a result of ill health. These may occur because of changes in employment status and a subsequent reduction of income. Many patients may find that they have to take long periods of time off work or are not able to return to work and may not be entitled to sick pay. The longer the patient is off work the more financial difficulties are likely to occur. Martin and Morgan (1975) found that 42% of those off work for one month had difficulties managing financially. The figure rose to 66% after one year.

Increased costs can also occur as a result of ill health. Many patients undergoing debilitating long term treatments will spend long periods at home incurring extra heating costs. Clear evidence has been found that extra costs exist on food, fuel and help in the home (*Disability, Household Income and Expenditure – Family Expenditure Survey*, 1990). Thus patients may find that they are not able to meet their normal financial commitments because of changes in income and outgoings as a result of ill-health. This may be particularly difficult to cope with at a time when the patient is having to deal with the stresses of a life-threatening illness.

3. RESOURCES

(1) The welfare adviser will have knowledge of the following.

    (a) The state benefits system.
    (b) Background to debt problems.
    (c) The working procedures of the Department of Social Security (DSS).
    (d) Specialist agencies which can give more complex advice.
    (e) Basic theory in relation to the impact of illness and crises.
    (f) Sources of funding.

(2) The welfare adviser will have skills in:

    (a) Communication – to give information and interpret it in a way understandable to the patient.
    (b) Teaching – to educate the patient on benefits and procedures of the DSS in assessing eligibility for benefits, and to educate medical staff on appropriate referrals.
    (c) Practical matters – to follow through benefit applications with patients, and to follow through procedures to alleviate financial difficulties if appropriate.

(3) There will be a system for referral and feedback to and from other members of the multidisciplinary team.

(4) The welfare adviser will have access to current technical information on benefits.

(5) Information leaflets will be available for patients and families.

(6) The welfare adviser will have access to professional continuing education.

(7) The welfare adviser will have access to a telephone and a suitable room in order to interview patients in confidence and privacy.

(8) The welfare adviser will have access to a range of current literature related to financial issues.

4. PROFESSIONAL PRACTICE

(1) The welfare adviser will:

   (a) Make an initial assessment of the financial problems that the patient perceives him/herself to have.
   (b) Obtain a comprehensive assessment of the patient's financial situation – income and outgoings.
   (c) Assess the patient's ability to follow any solution to the problem.

(2) The welfare adviser, together with the patient and family, will decide what course of action to take.

   (a) The patient will not be referred without his or her permission.
   (b) The patient will be helped to understand his or her financial situation.
   (c) The patient and the welfare adviser will look at income and outgoings and possible changes so that planning and negotiations can be undertaken in a manner which fosters the patient's and family's sense of control.
   (d) The welfare adviser will help the patient to find ways to maximize his or her income, including take-up of benefits for which he or she is eligible.
   (e) The welfare adviser will mediate between the patient and benefit agency to help minimize misunderstandings that may occur.
   (f) The welfare adviser will represent patient's interests and acquire services and benefits that are the patient's right but which the patient might not be able to negotiate for him/herself.
   (g) The welfare adviser will contact benefit agencies and advise patients on appeal procedures as appropriate.
   (i) The welfare adviser will negotiate with the patient's creditors.
   (j) The welfare adviser will negotiate with employers regarding sick pay arrangements.
   (k) The patient will be helped through the 'maze' when applying for benefits and negotiate with the DSS.

(3) The welfare adviser will:

   (a) Evaluate interventions and monitor follow-up; also pursue those initiatives carried out by the patient at regular periods as agreed with the patient.
   (b) Ensure that the patient understands the need for follow-up as above and will contact the welfare adviser as necessary.
   (c) Make case recordings and keep them in a safe and confidential place.

5. OUTCOMES

(1) The patient and family report that they were provided with appropriate practical help and information.

(2) The welfare adviser considers that he or she had access to resources needed and was able to follow the prescribed professional practice. He or she also reports that the patient and family were provided with appropriate practical help and information.

(3) The case records will show evidence that resources were used and professional practice followed to ensure that patients and families were provided with appropriate information, and given appropriate practical help in order to alleviate financial problems if possible.

REFERENCES

Disability, Household Income and Expenditure – Family Expenditure Survey. (1990) HMSO, London.

Martin, J. & Morgan, M. (1975) *Prolonged Sickness and the Return to Work.* HMSO, London.

STATUTORY SOCIAL WORK

1. STANDARD STATEMENT

Social workers are legally obliged to identify and assess risks to patients who are vulnerable on grounds of being under age, mentally ill, elderly or disabled and to help find solutions to their needs in the least intrusive and coercive way.

2. RATIONALE

The framework of statutory work is defined by four major pieces of legislation, the Children Act (1989), the Mental Health Act (1983), the Disabled Persons Act (1986) and the Community Care Act (1991).

(1) The Children Act (1989) commits local authorities and their social services departments to:

   (a) Identify children in need and provide services to help them achieve a reasonable standard of health and development.
   (b) Recognize the child's welfare as paramount in all court proceedings.
   (c) Promote the upbringing of children in need by their families and provide advice, guidance, counselling, home help and accommodation in partnership with the parents on the basis of clearly identified needs and written agreements.
   (d) Investigate if there is reasonable cause to suspect that a child is suffering or likely to suffer significant harm and to take appropriate steps to protect the child.

(2) The Mental Health Act (1983) invests part of the authority in applying for detention and assessment and/or compulsory treatment of psychiatrically disturbed patients in the role of the approved social worker. The sections of the Act can only be invoked if there is a clear need for psychiatric and social work assessment to establish the nature of disturbed behaviour or a need to treat an already diagnosed condition. With chronic mental illness, any proposed treatment must demonstrably be able to make a difference to the patient's condition. The approved social worker assesses, in co-operation with a psychiatrist and a second doctor, whether a patient:

   (a) Suffers from a mental illness and shows behaviour which constitutes a danger to him or herself or others.
   (b) Accepts treatment on a voluntary basis, preferably by community-based resources.
   (c) Having refused voluntary treatment, can be legally detained in hospital under the committal sections of the Act.

(3) Under the Disabled Persons Act (1986), local authorities identify disabled people and provide a range of services with a view to promoting independent living in the community, for example domiciliary care, provision of telephones, radio and TVs, recreational facilities, holidays and adaptations to the home.

(4) The Community Care Act (1991) stipulates the need to:

   (a) Promote the development of domiciliary, day and respite services to enable people to live in their own homes wherever feasible and sensible.
   (b) Ensure that service providers make support for carers a high priority.
   (c) Make proper assessment of need and good case management the cornerstone of high quality.

3. RESOURCES

(1) The social worker will have a good working knowledge of the following.

(a) Relevant legislation, social services departmental procedures and guidance issued by the Department of Health.
(b) Community resources generally available from local authorities under the provisions of relevant legislation.
(c) Indicators of child physical and sexual abuse and emotional neglect (Children Act, 1989).
(d) The process and purpose of multi-disciplinary investigation and assessment of 'significant harm' in relation to children (Children Act 1989).
(e) Symptoms of mental disturbance, psychiatric classifications and main treatment modalities (Mental Health Act 1983).
(f) Social work criteria for using committal sections (Mental Health Act 1983).
(g) Principles and practice of creating appropriate packages of care (Community Care Act 1991).
(h) Statutory, local authority and voluntary agency resources that will help patients and their carers to live independently in the community (Community Care Act 1991).
(i) Basic professional theory in relation to child development, family dynamics, impact of illness and crises.

(2) The social worker will have developed skills in the following.

(a) Identifying and assessing risks to children, mentally ill, elderly and disabled people.
(b) Assessing where family interaction is creating serious risks to one or more persons, and intervene in appropriate circumstances to reduce that risk and enable the family to make optimal use of its own resources.
(c) Engaging patient and/or family in work on the basis of shared goals to relieve the risk to vulnerable family members.
(d) Crisis intervention.
(e) Convening and facilitating multidisciplinary meetings.
(f) Communicating relevant information about a case with colleagues both within the hospital and in the community and providing, where necessary, for follow-up support for the patient.
(g) Educating other health care professionals about the key elements of relevant legislature and the local authority's role in community care.

(3) The social worker has to rely on the multidisciplinary team as the main source of referrals. The psychiatrist and lecturer/practitioner (psychological care) would act as primary collaborators in terms of mental health emergencies; paediatricians and community liaison nurses in terms of the Children Act. All paramedical and rehabilitation staff, ward-based nurses and community liaison nurses are resources in relation to community care and disability.

(4) There is written information available for patients and their families including the following.

(a) Community care plans for the residents of the local areas.
(b) A brochure explaining how a parent can appoint a legal guardian for his or her children.
(c) Explanation of the complaints procedure.
(d) File copies of the Children Act and the Mental Health Act.

(5) The social worker needs access to a quiet interview space conducive to discussion and respecting the privacy of patient, relatives and professionals.

4. PROFESSIONAL PRACTICE

(1) The social worker makes initial and ongoing assessment:

(a) Under the Children Act as to whether:

- there is a child in need
- the child or parents are eligible for local authority resources
- a child is 'suffering' or likely to 'suffer significant harm'.

(b) Under the Mental Health Act as to whether:

- the person is suffering from 'a mental disorder of a nature or degree to warrant detention for assessment (or assessment followed by medical treatment)'
- the person needs to be detained 'in the interests of his own health or safety or with a view to the protection of others'
- the person suffers from 'mental illness, severe mental impairment or psychopathic disorder of a nature or degree which makes it appropriate to receive treatment in hospital'.

(c) Under the Disabled Persons Act 1986 as to whether:

- the person is eligible for a range of services offered by the local authority to meet his or her needs.

(d) Under the Community Care Act 1991 as to:

- what services and information are available to help carers in their task
- eligibility for services which promote independent living.

(2) The social worker plans intervention in consultation and collaboration with the multidisciplinary team, and keeps the patient and family fully informed of the procedures and goals of the intervention where possible.

(a) Broad goals for statutory work under the Children Act are:

- to enable parents to plan for the care of their children after one parent's death
- to make available specialist legal advice, where necessary, to a parent to use the procedures of the Act to appoint a legal guardian
- to safeguard the wellbeing of children known to us, by supporting the family and to invoke legal powers as a last resort
- to involve parents and, if appropriate, members of the extended family in decision making
- to ascertain the child's wishes and plan with an understanding of the child's religious persuasion, racial origin, cultural and linguistic background.

(b) Broad goals for statutory work under the Mental Health Act are:

- to work towards voluntary acceptance of treatment, where appropriate
- to promote and protect the civil liberties of the patient
- to consult, as much as possible, with patient and relatives and to assess the patient's symptoms in a wider context

SOCIAL WORK

- to promote the use of community based resources (day centres, out-patient clinics, general practitioners, community psychiatric nurses) as far as possible.

(c) Broad goals for statutory work under the Disabled Persons Act (1986) and the Community Care Act (1991) are:

- to involve and support informal carers
- to promote independent living for elderly and disabled people, by an optimal use of community services.

5. OUTCOMES

(1) Patients report that their rights were considered and protected and that they are satisfied with the help they received from the social worker.

(2) The social worker reports that he or she had access to the resources needed and was able to follow the prescribed professional practice. The social worker also considers that patients' rights of were considered and protected through the least intrusive procedures possible.

(3) Documentation shows evidence that resources were used and professional practice followed to assist individuals in understanding the circumstance and that care was geared to their desires as much as possible.

REFERENCES

Department of Health, Home Office, Department of Education and Science, Welsh Office (1991) *Working Together*. HMSO, London.
Department of Health (1988) *Protecting Children*. HMSO, London.
Department of Health (1991a) *The Care of Children*. HMSO, London.
Department of Health (1991b) *The Children Act, 1989, Guidance and Regulations*, Vols 1–9. HMSO, London.

Acts of Parliament
Children Act, 1989.
Chronically Sick and Disabled Persons Act, 1970.
Community Care Act, 1991.
Disabled Persons Act, 1986.

WORKING WITH ADULT PATIENTS AND THEIR CHILDREN

1. STANDARD STATEMENT

Social work for parents aims to provide support and help in talking with their children in a clear and age appropriate manner about the implications of cancer, treatment and, if necessary, the possible death of the parent. Parents would also be offered help in planning realistic future care for their children.

2. RATIONALE

The impact of cancer is traumatic and stressful, and often invokes an intense response. Parents with cancer quite understandably want to protect their children from unnecessary emotional upset, but in so doing can easily exclude and isolate them. This leaves the children unsupported when they are trying to make sense of what is happening.

'For children as for adults, fantasies are often worse than the reality. They may fear catching the disease, or worry that they caused it by naughty behaviour; they need clear, simple and honest explanations'.

(Black, 1989)

A child may not understand about the nature of a parent's illness and prognosis and parents are often frightened about how the child will react. They worry that dealing with reality may damage the child. Sometimes, if the prognosis is poor, the adult is so angry or distressed about the impending loss that he or she is unable to talk constructively to the child about it.

'The adult may think that the children are too young, or too fragile, to handle direct information. Unfortunately this decision joins family members in a conspiracy of silence that deprives the child/ren of their rights to confront, question and resolve their grief.'

(Jewett, 1986)

Bowlby (1980), whose work on separation and attachment shaped our fundamental understanding of children and loss, believes that a child can resolve losses just as favourably as an adult, given the following conditions:

1. The child has enjoyed a reasonably secure relationship with his parents before the loss.
2. He receives prompt and accurate information about what has happened, and is allowed to ask all sorts of questions and have them answered as honestly as possible.
3. He participates in the family grieving, including funeral rites.
4. He has the comforting presence of a parent or adult whom he trusts and can rely on in a continuing relationship.

(Cited by Jewett, 1986. p. 3)

Ideally, children need preparation to cope with any changes brought about by the illness of a parent, and most especially before the death of a parent or relative. It is important that they have opportunities to ask questions and explore emotions. Children react to serious illness and death in many ways, some at once and some after considerable delay. They may deny that it is happening or be angry with others who 'allowed' it to happen. They may express anxiety and fear. Many children, for example when faced with losing a parent, will panic that the remaining parent will also become ill and die, or that they themselves have been instrumental through their behaviour and caused their parent to die. They need explicit, direct reassurance about what is happening and why.

Children sometimes upset adults by seeming callous, but this is part of their need to concentrate on the present and to explore their world. It does not mean that they do not feel sad. They also need to be able to make their own decisions about how involved they wish to be – whether they wish to be with the parent when dying, do they wish to see the body, go to the funeral, etc. It is important, therefore, that there have been clear explanations in advance of what will happen.

> '...there is now plenty of evidence that children can respond with a high degree of adaptability to painful emotional upsets if they are given the facts in a kind and careful way and given opportunities to ask questions and talk to the involved adults....'
>
> (Cooklin, 1989)

When a parent acknowledges that the illness is life-threatening, it is natural that he or she thinks about organizing appropriate child care provision in case 'the worst should happen'. Ideally parents should be helped early on to think through what concerns and wishes they have for their children's future. This is particularly true for a single parent if there is no obvious or suitable person to take over. But even where there is a surviving parent, the changes for the family are fundamental and potentially overwhelming. Because this is such a painful subject to contemplate, it is often not dwelt upon and not pursued to a conclusion. When a patient has been told, however, that a cure is not possible, it becomes essential that he or she is offered support to work through in detail the plans to be made for the care of the children. Experience suggests that the process of clarifying questions and thinking through possible plans not only has a positive outcome for the children in the long run, but also, importantly, reduces anxiety in the patient. Such planning also dramatically reduces the likelihood of statutory social service involvement at a moment of great crisis for the whole family.

---

3. RESOURCES

(1) A qualified social worker (Certificate of Qualification in Social Work or Diploma in Social Work) will have a baseline knowledge of the following.

   (a) Normal family functioning, life cycle events.
   (b) The impact of illness, loss and grief on adults and children.
   (c) Child development.
   (d) The impact of crisis on adults and children.
   (e) The main types of cancer and treatment and their potential side-effects (e.g. hair loss, nausea, fatigue, temporary memory impairment).
   (f) Child care legislation.
   (g) The skills of other appropriate disciplines in dealing with communication issues.

(2) The social worker will have developed skills in the following.

   (a) Assessing the process through which the family communicates about difficult issues.
   (b) Exploring the beliefs and values which underly the family's actions.
   (c) Ascertaining what the issues are and why they may currently be difficult to resolve.
   (d) Understanding family dynamics and working within a systemic or psychotherapeutic framework.
   (e) Helping parents and children to explore safe ways of resolving communication issues.
   (f) Defining concrete and achievable goals which are explicit for the worker and for the patient and family.
   (g) Communicating clearly with the multidisciplinary team what the focus of work is.
   (h) Working jointly with other professionals where the focus of the work needs their specific technical knowledge.
   (i) Working directly with children, if appropriate.

(3) The social worker depends upon members of the multidisciplinary team, primarily the ward-based nurses, to refer patients for assessment. Self-referrals by patient or relative are also possible. Referrals are also received from the lecturer/practitioner (psychological care).

(4) The social worker has knowledge and skills to work in partnership with children, parents and carers.

(5) The social worker has knowledge of and access to departmental procedures and the Department of Health guidance document *Working Together* (DoH 1991).

(6) There is a range of written information such as booklets, work books and literature for parents and children of all ages.

(7) The social worker will have access to a range of information and resources in the community.

(8) The social worker will have access to interview space that is large enough for meeting families, and protects the privacy of the patient as well as having an atmosphere conducive to discussion.

(9) The social worker will have an opportunity to develop professional skills and have access to departmental training on policy and procedures.

4. PROFESSIONAL PRACTICE

(1) The social worker makes an initial and ongoing assessment of the following.

(a) The response of the patient, family and child or children to previous stressful events and previous coping strategies.
(b) The degree to which shock and grief inhibit the capacity to cope.
(c) The specific blocks that are stopping communication at present.
(d) What the children know and what they would like or need to know.
(e) The larger context of which the communication difficulty is a part.
(f) Other problems that affect the communication difficulty (previous experience of cancer, illness, loss, grief, and changing roles within family, etc.)
(g) The patient and family's clarity about what the difficulty is and what they want to do about it.
(h) What information they might need to reduce unnecessary stress during hospitalization and treatment.
(i) Whether parents are confident in talking to children, whether they see the importance of sharing information and emotions about what is happening with other family members.
(j) How parental responsibilities are normally divided and what effect subsequent changes caused by the illness (physical appearance, reduced mobility, etc.) are having on each child.
(k) Whether they are able to plan appropriately for the future in full knowledge of regulations of the Children Act (1989) – for example, appointment of a legal guardian.
(l) Practical needs of children and family in terms of financial problems and help at home.

(2) The social worker plans help with the patient and child or family, and the multidisciplinary team.

(a) The patient and family agree to the referral prior to discussion with the social work department.

(b) The social worker subsequently:

- contacts the professional referrer to ascertain his or her assessment of the problem and who else is involved
- makes an initial assessment interview with those concerned to establish goals for work
- agrees on the number of sessions with the patient and family, and on how the agreed goals will be reviewed
- informs the multidisciplinary team of significant changes and records these in the patient's notes.

(3) The implementation of social work goals is monitored by the line manager through regular supervision where effectiveness can be evaluated. Monitoring of progress by the social worker is also an integral part of the therapeutic process.

(4) The social worker will assess the need for re-referral onto other disciplines for further help.

(5) If further help is needed by a child or patient upon discharge, the social worker (with the patient's permission) sends a case work summary to professionals in the community outlining the areas of concern for follow-up.

5. OUTCOMES

(1) The patient reports that he or she has found a way to talk about cancer issues with his or her children and is satisfied with the help offered by the social worker.

(2) The social worker will report that the family was offered options and that with these they were able to discuss issues in a way that is constructive for the children and for the adults.

(3) Documentation will show that resources were used and professional practice followed to facilitate the parent to explore ways to talk with the children about current issues in clear and age-appropriate ways.

REFERENCES

Black, D. (1989) Life-threatening illness, children and family therapy. *Journal of Family Therapy*, **11**, 81–101.

Bowlby, J. (1980) *Attachment and Loss*, Volumes 1, 2, 3, Hogarth Press, London.

Cooklin, A. (1989) Tenderness and toughness in the face of distress. *Palliative Medicine*, **3**, 89–95.

Department of Health (1991) *Working Together Under The Children Act 1985*. HMSO, London.

Jewett, C. (1986) *Helping Children Cope with Separation and Loss*, Batsford Academic, London.

Standards of Care

Speech and Language Therapy

GENERAL STANDARD FOR ACCESS TO SPEECH AND LANGUAGE THERAPY

1. STANDARD STATEMENT

Speech and langauge therapy is directed towards the assessment, differential diagnosis and management of communication and swallowing difficulties arising from cancer and/or its treatment.

2. RESOURCES

(1) A practising member of the College of Speech and Language Therapists will be available to assess, diagnose and treat where appropriate.

(2) The speech and language therapist will have access to ongoing education/support. The members of the department will be responsible for the collation and dissemination of information and experience and for arranging department-based teaching sessions.

(3) A referral system will be in operation as follows.

    (a) Speech and language therapists take both written and verbal referrals from all members of the multidisciplinary health care team. Speech therapists may also take patient/carers referrals.

    (b) Speech and language therapists regularly visit head and neck, neurology and paediatric units, to exchange information and receive referrals.

    (c) Referrals can be sent to the speech and language therapy department or telephoned in before 5.00 PM. In the case of an urgent referral a speech therapist can be bleeped.

    (d) Speech and language therapists attend specialist clinics in order to screen for patients with speech therapy needs and give advice as appropriate.

    (e) Speech and language therapists attend multidisciplinary ward meetings to collect referrals.

    (f) Speech and language therapists carry bleeps in order that they may be contacted easily.

    (g) The speech and language therapist will see pre-operative laryngectomy and glossectomy cases on admission. Urgent dysphagia cases are assessed within 24 hours of receipt of the referral. Other referrals received will be dealt with as soon as possible.

(4) An out-patient appointment system will be in operation as follows.

    (a) All patients referred for out-patient speech and language therapy will be contacted within one week of receipt of the referral to arrange an appropriate appointment time.

    (b) Out-patients may attend for speech and language therapy between 10 AM and 4 PM Monday to Friday, the time and frequency of these treatments will be decided by the speech and language therapist taking up the referral.

(5) A referral system to other speech and language therapy departments or other members of the multidisciplinary team will be in operation as follows.

    (a) All members of the multidisciplinary health care team will take both written and verbal referrals from speech and language therapists. These will be documented in the speech therapy notes.

    (b) All referrals to other speech therapy departments should be in writing with a copy filed in the speech therapy notes.

(6) 'Feedback' system to the referrer will be in operation. Verbal or written feedback is given to the referring health care professional on completion of assessment. A copy of all written reports is filed in the speech therapy notes.

(7) The speech and language therapist will have access to medical information about all patients with speech therapy needs.

(8) Other members of the multidisciplinary team will be available to act as a resource and source of referral to the patient, family and speech and language therapist.

(9) A range of 'standards of care' for specialist areas of speech and language therapy practice will be available to speech and language therapy staff.

(10) A range of speech therapy advice and information sheets will be available for patients.

(11) A range of aids and equipment and a system for the loaning of this equipment will be available.

(12) A speech and language therapy department will be available including:

- an ENT equipped out-patient cubicle
- a designated treatment area to offer patients privacy and quiet
- office accommodation where notes and equipment may be kept securely and staff may carry out paperwork
- storage facilities.

(13) The speech and language therapist will have access to clerical assistance.

(14) The speech and language therapist will have available a documentation system to record professional practice.

3. PROFESSIONAL PRACTICE

(1) The speech and language therapist undertakes an assessment, analyses the assessment and makes a differential diagnosis of the patient's speech therapy condition.

(2) Following the diagnosis the speech and language therapist agrees to a plan of management with the patient and family which may involve specific treatment programmes where appropriate.

(3) The speech and language therapist implements the management plan in conjunction with the patient, family and other members of the multidisciplinary team.

(4) The speech and language therapist evaluates the effectiveness of the plan by reassessing the patient, and adjusts interventions according to subjective and objective changes in the patient's condition.

(5) The speech and language therapist liaises and co-ordinates such interventions with other members of the multidisciplinary team and/or other speech therapy departments to ensure that the optimum level of care is achieved and that continuity of care on discharge is facilitated.

(6) The speech and language therapist documents all aspects of professional practice in the departmental records and, where appropriate, records speech therapy treatment/intervention in the medical and/or nursing notes.

4. OUTCOMES

(1) The patient and family report that the patient achieved his or her maximum potential of communication and swallowing function. They also report that they understood the long term management of any residual disability or dysfunction and that they were satisfied with the care received.

(2) The speech and language therapist considers that he or she had access to the resources as listed and was able to follow the described professional practice. The speech therapist also reports that the patient achieved maximum potential of communication and swallowing function and understood the long term management of any residual disability or dysfunction.

(3) The documentation system shows evidence that resources were used and professional practice followed in order for the patient to achieve his or her maximum potential of communication and swallowing function. There will be evidence that the patient and family understood the long term management of any residual disability or dysfunction and were satisfied with the care given.

STANDARD FOR PATIENTS EXPERIENCING DYSPHAGIA

1. STANDARD STATEMENT

Speech and language therapy for patients who are experiencing difficulties with swallowing is directed towards enabling the patient to achieve maximum swallowing potential and facilitating adaptation to this disability.

2. RATIONALE

Dysphagia is difficulty in transferring solids or liquids from the oral cavity to the stomach. The normal swallow requires an intact anatomy with normal mucosa and neuromuscular function, and in patients with cancer the dysphagia may be directly caused by the malignant process, by its treatment or may be a consequence of associated conditions (Regnard, 1987).

Patients with cancer presenting with dysphagia are most frequently found in the head and neck and neuro-oncology clinical populations. Paediatric oncology patients may be similarly affected. Aird *et al.* (1983), for example, found that 38% of their series of patients with head and neck cancer suffered from dysphagia. Robertson and Hornibrook (1982) found that 43% of their series presented with dysphagia, while 83% would eventually suffer from dysphagia.

Figures for the neuro-oncology population are difficult to find but tumours are well known to cause damage to the cranial nerves or, for instance, to arise directly in the brain stem. Additionally any neurosurgery for malignancy could result in haemorrhage and dysphagia from cerebro-vascular accident.

It is widely accepted that dysphagia necessitates a multidisciplinary team approach for the safe evaluation and treatment of patients with a swallowing problem that makes oral feeding difficult or impossible (Logemann, 1983). The speech and language therapist plays a key role in the assessment, planning and co-ordination of care.

3. RESOURCES

(1) A practising member of the College of Speech and Language Therapists is available to assess, advise and treat where appropriate.

(2) The speech and language therapist will have completed a minimum of three days formal post-graduate training in dysphagia.

(3) The speech and language therapist will have a knowledge of the following.

    (a) The effects of cancer and/or its treatment upon the ability to swallow.
    (b) The position paper on dysphagia prepared by the College of Speech Therapists (April 1990).
    (c) The normal swallowing mechanism.
    (d) Reading and interpreting videoflouroscopy films.
    (e) The signs and symptoms of aspiration.
    (f) Tracheostomy tubes – their availability and indications for use.

(4) The speech and language therapist will have skills in:

    (a) Communication – to convey a sensitive and empathetic attitude, and to gain the confidence of the patient and family.

(b) Teaching – to teach the patient compensatory swallowing techniques.
(c) Practical techniques – in the preparation of foods.

(5) The speech and language therapist will have access to on-going education/support. The members of the department will be responsible for the collation and dissemination of information and experience and for arranging department-based teaching sessions.

(6) The speech and language therapist will provide ongoing education and support for other professionals involved in dysphagia management.

(7) A system will be available for other members of the multidisciplinary team to refer patients experiencing dysphagia (see page 183). For cases of dysphagia the referral needs to be accompanied by written medical confirmation.

(8) A referral system to other speech and language therapy departments or other members of the multidisciplinary team will be in operation as follows.

(a) All members of the multidisciplinary health care team will take both written and verbal referrals from speech therapists. These will be documented in the speech therapy notes.
(b) All referrals to other speech and language therapy departments should be in writing with a copy filed in the speech therapy notes.

(9) 'Feedback' system to the referrer will be in operation. Verbal or written feedback is given to the referring health care professional on completion of assessment. A copy of all written reports is filed in the speech therapy notes.

(10) The speech and language therapist will have access to medical information about patients experiencing dysphagia.

(11) Other members of the multidisciplinary team will be available to act as a resource and source of referral to the patient, family and speech and language therapist including medical staff, nursing staff, dietitian and oral hygienist.

(12) A range of aids and equipment will be available. The speech and language therapists have access to diagnostic radiology departments including videofluoroscopy. Referral for radiological investigation of dysphagia will require a signature from a member of the medical staff.

(13) Written information will be available for the patient and/or family (e.g. *Patient Information Series* Booklet No. 7 and dysphagia instruction sheets).

(14) Local policies on safety procedures will be available to the speech and language therapist (e.g. relating to cross infection, use of suction, health and safety recommendations for staff etc.)

(15) The speech and language therapist will have access to clerical assistance.

(16) The speech and language therapist will have available a documentation system to record professional practice.

4. PROFESSIONAL PRACTICE

(1) The speech and language therapist will have appropriate indemnity cover provided by the College of Speech and Language Therapists. The speech and language therapists

will have overall responsibility for the speech therapy input to the team with which they are involved.

(2) The speech and language therapist makes an initial and ongoing assessment of the following.

    (a) The patient's pattern of swallowing.
    (b) The possible risks of aspiration.
    (c) The patient's nutritional status and fluid intake.
    (d) The patient's and family's needs for information and support regarding dysphagia.

(3) The speech and language therapist analyses the assessment and agrees to a plan of treatment with team, the patient and family.

    ● **NB** Where the medical team chooses a course of action which in the opinion of the speech and language therapist is harmful to the patient, he or she discusses this with the medical team. Withdrawal of involvement may be considered and such action is accompanied by a written explanation.

(4) The speech and language therapist implements the management plan in conjunction with the patient, family and other members of the multidisciplinary team.

    (a) The patient is offered information and teaching of exercises to assist the oropharyngeal musculature, enabling him or her to regain a pattern of swallowing.
    (b) The patient and family are offered information and advice regarding the choice and preparation of food.
    (c) The speech and language therapist offers intensive treatment where appropriate.

(5) The speech and language therapist evaluates the effectiveness of the plan by reassessing the patient, and adjusts interventions according to subjective and objective changes in the patient's condition.

(6) The speech and language therapist liaises and co-ordinates such interventions with other members of the multidisciplinary team and/or other speech and language therapy departments to ensure that the optimum level of care is achieved and that continuity of care on discharge is facilitated. Where necessary the speech and language therapist negotiates the delegation of certain tasks to other members of the team, who are then regarded as 'proxy therapists'.

    ● **NB** The speech and language therapists remain responsible for the proxy intervention if a task is delegated. The proxy therapists are required to abide by the guidelines with regard to the procedure involved and documentation.

(7) The decision to discharge a patient from speech therapy is discussed with the remainder of the team, the patient and the family. It is possible that overall discharge from the hospital may be delayed in dysphagic patients who have not made sufficient progress to manage safely at home.

(8) The speech and language therapist documents all aspects of professional practice in the departmental records and, where appropriate, records speech therapy treatment and intervention in the medical and/or nursing notes.

(9) Speech and language therapy students will be directly supervised at all times by an appropriately skilled and experienced speech and language therapist when involved in the assessment and/or treatment of dysphagic patients.

5. OUTCOMES

(1) The patient and family report that the patient achieved his or her maximum potential swallowing function and that they understood the long term management of any residual disability or dysfunction. They also report that their needs for information and practical support were met and that they were satisfied with the care received.

(2) The speech and language therapist considers that he or she had access to the resources as listed and was able to follow the described professional practice. The speech therapist also reports that the patient achieved his or her maximum potential swallowing function and understood the long term management of any residual disability or dysfunction. The speech and language therapist also considers that the patient and family's needs for information and practical support were met.

(3) The documentation system will show evidence that resources were used and professional practice followed in order that the patient achieved their maximum potential of swallowing function and that the patient and family understood the long term management of any residual disability or dysfunction. There will be evidence that the patient and family's needs for information and for practical care were met and that they were satisfied with the care given.

REFERENCES

Aird, D. C., Bihan, J. & Smith, C. (1982) Clinical problems in the continuing care of head and neck Cancer patients. *Ear Nose & Throat Journal*, **62**, 334.

College of Speech Therapists, Dysphagia Working Party (1990) *Position Paper (April 1990) – Dysphagia*. College of Speech Therapists, London.

Logemann, J. (1983) *Evaluation and Treatment of Swallowing Disorders*. College Hill Press, San Diego, California.

Regnard, C. F. B. (1987) Contemporary palliation of difficult symptoms. In *Baillière's Clinical Oncology*, Vol. I (No. 2) Chapter 5. Baillière-Tindall, Eastbourne.

Robertson, M. S. & Hornibrook, J. (1982) The presenting symptoms of head and neck cancer. *New Zealand Medical Journal*, **95**, 708.

STANDARD FOR PATIENTS UNDERGOING LARYNGECTOMY

1. STANDARD STATEMENT

Speech and language therapy for the patient undergoing laryngectomy aims to ensure the patient has a clear understanding of the anatomical and physiological changes involved, that the patient is aware of the long term options for communication and that help is offered for any swallowing difficulties which might arise.

2. RATIONALE

Laryngectomy is the surgical removal of the 'voice box' or larynx. Cancer of the larynx represents 2.09% of all cancers (S E Thames Cancer Registry, 1988). Rehabilitation for the laryngectomee involves offering a means of producing voice in an alternative way. The speech and language therapist plays a key role in promoting the patient's understanding, and pre-operative involvement is therefore strongly recommended to assess the patient's communication skills and adjustments to diagnosis (Edels, 1985, Evans, 1990).

The elements of communication include speech, language and voice. Voice can be defined as the sound produced when expiratory airflow from the lungs travels up through the larynx under pressure, and this causes the vocal folds to vibrate. This sound is then modified by the articulators, the ora-pharyngeal tract and nasal resonance. The laryngectomee will no longer have the means to produce this sound. A proportion of laryngectomy patients will spontaneously develop oesophageal voice but the success rate for gaining functional voice is low. Hence, surgical voice restoration is offered to the vast majority of patients at the hospital.

3. RESOURCES

(1) A practising member of the College of Speech and Language Therapists will be available to assess, diagnose and treat where appropriate.

(2) The speech and language therapist will have a knowledge of the following.

    (a) Oncology and the effects of the disease and its treatment upon the post-operative status of the laryngectomee i.e. its effects on communication and swallowing.
    (b) The elements of communication.
    (c) The mechanisms of voice production.
    (d) Alternative means of voice production.
    (e) The principles, sizing, fitting and use of voice protheses (valves), which is obtained through practical postgraduate training.
    (f) The management of voice valve emergencies.

(3) The speech and language therapist will have skills in:

    (a) Communication – to discuss speech therapy intervention with the patient and family and to gain their trust and co-operation.
    (b) Teaching – to demonstrate the principles, cleaning and use of the valve with the patient and/or family.
    (c) Practical techniques – valve fitting and to undertake trouble-shooting where appropriate.

(4) The speech and language therapist will have access to ongoing education and support. The members of the department will be responsible for the collation and dissemination of information and experience and for arranging department-based teaching sessions.

(5) A system will be in operation for other members of the multidisciplinary team to refer patients pre-operatively (see page 183).

(6) A referral system to other speech and language therapy departments or other members of the multidisciplinary team will be in operation as follows.

  (a) All members of the multidisciplinary health care team will take both written and verbal referrals from speech and language therapists. These will be documented in the speech therapy notes.

  (b) All referrals to other speech and language therapy departments should be in writing with a copy filed in the speech therapy notes.

(7) 'Feedback' system to the referrer will be in operation as follows. Verbal or written feedback is given to the referring health care professional on completion of assessment. A copy of all written reports is filed in the speech therapy notes.

(8) The speech and language therapist will have access to medical information about patients undergoing laryngectomy.

(9) Other members of the multidisciplinary team will be available to act as a resource and source of referral to the patient, family and speech and language therapist.

(10) The speech and language therapist will have access to the following range of practical equipment:

  - ENT lighting equipment and head mirror
  - protective spectacles/gloves/apron
  - metal instruments (e.g. curved forceps which can be sterilized satisfactorily)
  - adequate supplies of replacement voice valves and related items.

(11) Written instructions about coping with valve emergencies and cleaning procedures, will be given to the other health care professionals, the patient and the family.

(12) The speech and language therapist will have available written information for the patient and their family (e.g. the Royal Marsden Hospital *Patient Information Booklet 6: Laryngectomy, Your Questions Answered*, and instructions and diagrams from the speech therapy department).

(13) The speech and language therapist will have access to clerical help and office equipment, including a telephone.

(14) The speech and language therapist will have available a documentation system to record professional practice.

4. PROFESSIONAL PRACTICE

(1) The speech and language therapist makes an initial pre-operative and ongoing assessment of the following.

(a) The patient's communication skills.
(b) The patient's motivation and adjustments to diagnosis.
(c) The patient's body awareness, vision, hearing and dexterity.

(2) The speech and language therapist analyses the assessment and agrees to a plan of management with the patient and family.

(3) The speech and language therapist implements the management plan in conjunction with the patient, family and other members of the multidisciplinary team.

(a) The speech and language therapist offers the patient and family an explanation of his or her role in voice and swallowing rehabilitation.
(b) The speech and language therapist offers the patient and family information and explanation related to the anatomical and physiological changes necessitated by a laryngectomy and the subsequent effects this will have on communication and swallowing in language tailored to their individual capabilities.
(c) Post-operatively the speech and language therapist monitors the patient's progress, offering information, advice and communication charts where appropriate to the patient and family.
(d) The speech and language therapist undertakes the sizing and fitting of the patient's voice prosthesis in out-patients, and consults with medical colleagues for advice and/or practical help where indicated.
(e) The speech and language therapist offers intensive training as required in the cleaning and use of the voice valve, including offering instruction and teaching to the patient's family or carer if appropriate and also the nurse allocated to that patient.
(f) The speech and language therapist offers the patient and family continued individualized teaching, information and supervision as necessary.
(g) The speech and language therapist monitors the patient's progress using the voice valve at outpatient clinics, offering additional speech therapy if necessary.

(4) The speech and language therapist evaluates the effectiveness of the plan by reassessing the patient and adjusts interventions according to subjective and objective changes in the patient's condition.

(5) The speech and language therapist liaises and co-ordinates such interventions with other members of the multidisciplinary team and/or other speech therapy departments to ensure that the optimum level of care is achieved and that continuity of care on discharge is facilitated.

(6) The speech and language therapist documents all aspects of professional practice in the departmental records and, where appropriate, records speech therapy treatment and intervention in the medical and/or nursing notes.

(7) Following discussion with other members of the multidisciplinary team, the speech and language therapist may, if deemed appropriate, terminate speech therapy.

5. OUTCOMES

(1) The patient and family report that the patient achieved a level of communication acceptable to the patient and that their communication needs were met at a practical level and at an information/support level.

(2) The speech and language therapist considers that he or she had access to the resources as listed and was able to follow the described professional practice. The speech and language therapist also reports that the patient's communication (and possibly swallowing) needs have been met according to the criteria for referral and pre- and post-operative assessment, and that the patient is able to communicate at the optimum level feasible.

(3) The documentation system will show evidence that resources were used and professional practice followed in order for the patient's communication (and possibly swallowing) needs to be met according to the criteria for referral and pre- and post-operative assessment. The documentation system will also show that the patient is able to communicate at the optimum level feasible according to anatomical, physiological and psychological constraints. There will also be evidence that the patient and family feel that communication needs have been met at a practical level and at an information/support level.

REFERENCES

Edels, Y. (1985) *Laryngectomy: Diagnosis to Rehabilitation*. Croom Helm, London.
Evans, E. (1990) *Working with Laryngectomees*. Winslow Press, Bicester.

PART THREE

AUDITING TOOLS

Chaplaincy Standards of Care

SPIRITUAL NEEDS
PATIENT OPINION

The chaplains at The Royal Marsden Hospital are constantly trying to improve the service they provide to patients. It is of enormous help to have the views of patients to help us do this and we would like to collect some information from you about your experience of the care the chaplains have provided.

We would be very grateful if you would be willing to complete this questionnaire and return it in the envelope provided. The information you provide is confidential and will be treated accordingly.

Thank you for taking the time to complete this questionnaire

1. If you wanted to see a chaplain, do you consider that it was easy to contact him/her?   [ ] Yes [ ] No

   If no, what made it difficult?

2. When you did ask to see the chaplain, do you consider that he/she responded promptly?   [ ] Yes [ ] No

   If no, how long did you have to wait?

3. Did you find the services of the chaplain helpful?   [ ] Yes [ ] No

   What would have made them more helpful?

   What was most helpful?

4. Overall, were you satisfied with the services provided by the chaplains?   [ ] Yes [ ] No

   If no, what would have made you more satisfied?

   Do you have any other comments you would like to make?

Thank you once again for completing this questionnaire

SPIRITUAL NEEDS
CHAPLAIN OPINION

STANDARD STATEMENT

The aims of the chaplaincy for patients and their relatives who are experiencing spiritual distress are to facilitate and empower individuals in their search for meaning and purpose in life.

1. Do you consider that the ward staff were co-operative in making your services known to the patients? [ ] Yes [ ] No

If no, from whom did you not receive co-operation and why?

2. Do you consider that the referral
(a) Was made at an appropriate time? [ ] Yes [ ] No
(b) Was thoroughly and clearly communicated? [ ] Yes [ ] No

If no, please comment as to what was inappropriate or poorly communicated:

3. If part of your services included a recommendation that was dependent on a member of the multidisciplinary team, did the health care professional follow through on your recommendation? [ ] Yes [ ] No
[ ] Not
applicable

If no, why was the recommendation not carried out?

4. Do you consider that you had access to all the members of the multidisciplinary team that you required to achieve this standard? [ ] Yes [ ] No

If no, who was not available, and how did this impact on the care you were aiming to provide?

5. Do you consider that you had access to the equipment necessary to achieve this standard? [ ] Yes [ ] No

If no, what was not available and why?

6. Do you consider that you had access to the environment necessary to achieve this standard? [ ] Yes [ ] No

If no, what was unavailable or unsuitable and why?

7. Do you consider that you had access to the educational and managerial support necessary to achieve this standard?
Educational support [ ] Yes [ ] No
Managerial support [ ] Yes [ ] No

If no, what aspect(s) were not met and how did this impact on the care you were aiming to provide?

8. Do you feel that you were able to follow the professional practice described in the standard?   [ ] Yes [ ] No

If no, which sections were you unable to follow and why?

9. Do you consider that everything was offered to the patient to assist them in achieving their maximal spiritual integrity?   [ ] Yes [ ] No

If no, why?

10. Do you consider that the patient and/or family member achieved their maximal spiritual integrity?
Patient   [ ] Yes [ ] No
Family   [ ] Yes [ ] No

If no, please comment on why it was not achieved

11. Do you consider that the patient was satisfied with the care you provided?   [ ] Yes [ ] No

If no, why do you feel that the patient was not satisfied?

12. Overall, do you feel satisfied with the care that you delivered to the patient?   [ ] Yes [ ] No

If no, why were you not satisfied?

Are there any other comments you would like to make?

SPIRITUAL NEEDS
WARD STAFF OPINION

STANDARD STATEMENT

The aims of the chaplaincy for patients and their relatives who are experiencing spiritual distress are to facilitate and empower individuals in their search for meaning and purpose in life.

1. Did you have any difficulties contacting the chaplaincy? [ ] Yes [ ] No

Please comment as to what made it easy or difficult:

2. Once you contacted the chaplain, did he/she respond within a negotiated time? [ ] Yes [ ] No

If no, how did this impact on the care you were aiming to provide?

3. When you contacted the chaplain, did you find him/her helpful to you in your ability to care for the patient? [ ] Yes [ ] No

What did you find most helpful?

What would make them more helpful?

4. Do you consider that your contact with the chaplain better prepared you to deal with a similar situation/problem should it arise again? [ ] Yes [ ] No

What would better assist you?

5. Overall, are you satisfied with the services the chaplains provide related to meeting the patient's spiritual needs? [ ] Yes [ ] No

What do you consider would improve the service offered?

Are there any other comments you would like to make?

Dietetic Standards of Care

GENERAL STANDARD
PATIENT OPINION

The dietetic staff at The Royal Marsden Hospital are constantly trying to improve the service they provide for patients. It is of enormous help to have the views of patients to help us do this and we would like to collect some information from you about your experience of the care the dietitians have provided.

We would be very grateful if you would be willing to complete this questionnaire and return it in the envelope provided. The information you provide is confidential and will be treated accordingly.

Thank you for taking the time to complete this questionnaire

1. Were you clear about why the dietitian was asked to see you?   [ ] Yes [ ] No

   Please comment if you would like to:

2. Did you find the dietitian helpful?   [ ] Yes [ ] No

   If no, what could he/she have done to be more helpful?

3. If the dietitian made suggestions about your diet, were you able to   [ ] Yes [ ] No
   follow them while on the ward?

   If no, what made it difficult?

4. If you need to make changes in your diet when you go home, have
   you received enough guidance and practical information to do
   this?
   Guidance   [ ] Yes [ ] No
   Practical information   [ ] Yes [ ] No

   If no, what would have been more helpful?

5. If you were given written information about your diet, was it   [ ] Yes [ ] No
   helpful?   [ ] Did not
   receive any
   If not, what would have made it more helpful?

DIETETIC

6. Overall, do you feel satisfied with the care and information that the dietitian provided?

Care   [ ] Yes   [ ] No

Information   [ ] Yes   [ ] No

If no, what could have been done that would have made you feel more satisfied?

7. What did you find most helpful about the dietitian's care?

8. What did you find least helpful about the dietitian's care?

Are there any other comments that you would like to make?

Thank you once again for completing this questionnaire

GENERAL STANDARD
DIETITIAN OPINION

STANDARD STATEMENT

Dietetic care for patients requiring nutritional support is directed towards enabling patients to achieve their optimum nutritional status.

1. Do you consider that you had access to all the members of the multidisciplinary team that you required to achieve this standard? [ ] Yes [ ] No

   If no, who was not available, and how did this impact on the care you were aiming to provide?

2. Do you consider that you had access to the equipment necessary to achieve this standard? [ ] Yes [ ] No

   If no, what was not available and why?

3. Do you consider that you had access to the environment necessary to achieve this standard? [ ] Yes [ ] No

   If no, what was unavailable or unsuitable and why?

4. Do you consider that you had access to the educational and managerial support necessary to achieve this standard?
   Educational support [ ] Yes [ ] No
   Managerial support [ ] Yes [ ] No

   If no, what aspect(s) were lacking and how did this impact on the care you were providing?

5. Do you feel that you were able to follow the professional practice described in the standard? [ ] Yes [ ] No

   If no, which sections were you unable to follow and why?

6. Did you feel that you received co-operation and assistance from the other members of the multidisciplinary team? [ ] Yes [ ] No

   If no, who did you not receive co-operation from, and why?

7. Did you feel that the ward staff carried out your instructions as you requested? [ ] Yes [ ] No

   If no, who did not carry out the requests and why do you feel this was?

DIETETIC

8. Did you feel the patient's nutritional intake achieved an optimal level?   [ ] Yes   [ ] No

If no, what do you consider the reasons for this were?

9. Do you consider that the patient was satisfied with her treatment for this problem?   [ ] Yes   [ ] No

If no, why do you feel that the patient was not satisfied?

10. Overall, do you feel satisfied with the care that you delivered to the patient?   [ ] Yes   [ ] No

If no, why were you not satisfied?

Are there any other comments what you would like to make?

GENERAL STANDARD
DOCUMENTATION

| STANDARD STATEMENT |

Dietetic care for patients requiring nutritional support is directed towards enabling patients to achieve their optimum nutritional status.

Questions 1–2 relate to the dietetic department record card:

1. Is there evidence that the following were assessed?
   (a) Patient intake [ ] Yes [ ] No
   (b) Weight status [ ] Yes [ ] No
   (c) Nutritional requirements [ ] Yes [ ] No

2. Was the patient assessed for all the items listed in the standard of care? [ ] Yes [ ] No

   If not, which were omitted?

Questions 3–9 relate to the nursing care plan as the source of documentation.

3. Was the problem/area of care clearly stated and dated?
   Stated [ ] Yes [ ] No
   Dated [ ] Yes [ ] No

4. Were the goals/aims of nutritional care clearly stated? [ ] Yes [ ] No
   [ ] Not documented

5. Was the plan of action/programme of nutritional care clearly stated? [ ] Yes [ ] No
   [ ] Not documented

6. If the dietitian was contacted by the nursing staff, was there evidence that appropriate action was taken by the dietitian? [ ] Yes [ ] No
   [ ] Not applicable

7. Was there evidence of weekly evaluation by the dietitian? [ ] Yes [ ] No

8. If the patient required nutritional support or help at home, is there evidence that a plan was established to meet these needs? [ ] Yes [ ] No
   [ ] Not applicable

DIETETIC

9. If either of the following situations arose, is there evidence that this was documented by the dietitian in the medical notes?

(a) The medical staff made an inappropriate written referral [ ] Yes [ ] No

(b) Dietetic advice advocating TPN or tube feeding was not accepted by medical staff [ ] Yes [ ] No

Nursing Standards of Care

CHRONIC PAIN
PATIENT OPINION

The nursing staff of The Royal Marsden Hospital are constantly trying to improve the service it provides to patients. It is of enormous help to have the views of patients to help us do this and we would like to collect some information from you about your experience of the care the nurses have provided.

We would be very grateful if you would be willing to complete this questionnaire and return it in the envelope provided. The information you provide is confidential and will be treated accordingly.

Thank you for taking the time to complete this questionnaire

1. Do you feel that everything possible was done to control your pain? [ ] Yes [ ] No

If no, what else could have been done to help?

2. Did you have the opportunity to talk with the nurse about the cause of your pain? [ ] Yes [ ] No

Please comment if you would like to:

3. Did you have an opportunity to talk to the nurse about possible treatments for your pain? [ ] Yes [ ] No

Please comment if you would like to:

4. Did the nurse answer your questions adequately? [ ] Yes [ ] No

Please comment if you would like to:

5. Did you feel that the nursing staff had an understanding of the pain that you experienced? [ ] Yes [ ] No

Please comment if you would like to:

6. If a pain chart was used, did you find it helpful? [ ] Yes [ ] No

If no, why was it not helpful?

7. Did you feel that the side effects that you may have experienced [ ] Yes [ ] No
from taking a pain killer were clearly explained?

Please comment if you would like to:

8. Did you feel that your pain was reduced while in the hospital? [ ] Yes [ ] No

Please comment if you would like to:

Did you feel that your pain was relieved while you were in [ ] Yes [ ] No
hospital?

Please comment if you would like to:

9. Overall, do you feel satisfied with the care you received to control [ ] Yes [ ] No
your pain?

If no, please comment as to why you were not satisfied:

10. What did you find most helpful about the care you received?

11. What did you find the least helpful about the care you received for
your pain?

Have you any more comments that you would like to make?

Thank you once again for completing this questionnaire

CHRONIC PAIN
NURSE OPINION

STANDARD STATEMENT

Patients who are experiencing chronic pain(s) will receive nursing care directed towards controlling or relieving this symptom to achieve optimum quality of life for each individual patient.

1. Do you consider that you had access to all the members of the multidisciplinary team that you required to achieve this standard?   [ ] Yes   [ ] No

   If not, how did this impact on the care you were aiming to provide?

2. Do you consider that you had access to the equipment necessary to achieve this standard?   [ ] Yes   [ ] No

   If no, what was not available and why?

3. Do you consider that you had access to the environment necessary to achieve this standard?   [ ] Yes   [ ] No

   If no, what was unavailable or unsuitable, and why?

4. Do you consider that you had access to the educational and managerial support necessary to achieve this standard?
   Educational support   [ ] Yes   [ ] No
   Managerial   [ ] Yes   [ ] No

   If no, what aspect(s) were not met – and how did this impact on the care you were able to give?

5. Do you feel that you were able to follow the professional practice described in the standard?   [ ] Yes   [ ] No

   If no, which sections were you unable to follow and why?

6. Do you consider that you received adequate information (via report, care plans and documentation) to maintain continuity of care while caring for this patient?   [ ] Yes   [ ] No

   If no, what information were you lacking?

7. Do you consider that the patient had sufficient understanding to take their analgesic safely?   [ ] Yes   [ ] No

8. Do you consider that the patient's pain was minimized?   [ ] Yes   [ ] No

   Do you consider that the patient's pain was relieved?   [ ] Yes   [ ] No

   If no, why do you feel this was not the outcome?

NURSING

9. If you did not use a pain chart, why did you find it inappropriate?

10. Which non-pharmacological methods of pain control did you consider?

11. Do you consider that overall the patient was satisfied with his/her treatment for this problem?   [ ] Yes [ ] No

    If no, why do you feel that the patient was not satisfied?

12. Overall, do you feel satisfied with the care that you delivered to the patient?   [ ] Yes [ ] No

    If no, why were you not satisfied?

    Are there any other comments you would like to make?

CHRONIC PAIN DOCUMENTATION

> ### STANDARD STATEMENT

Patients who are experiencing chronic pain(s) will receive nursing care directed towards controlling or relieving this symptom to achieve optimum quality of life for each individual patient.

1. Is there evidence that the patient was assessed for:
    (a) Types of pain   [ ] Yes   [ ] No
    (b) Location of pain(s)   [ ] Yes   [ ] No
    (c) Alleviating factors   [ ] Yes   [ ] No
    (d) Aggravating factors   [ ] Yes   [ ] No
    (e) History of analgesic use   [ ] Yes   [ ] No
    (f) Effectiveness of previous analgesia   [ ] Yes   [ ] No

2. Were the patient's needs identified in the assessment addressed in the plan?   [ ] Yes   [ ] No

    If not, which were omitted?

3. Were the outcomes based on realistic progression (e.g. pain free at sleep, rest and movement)?   [ ] Yes   [ ] No

4. Is there evidence of reassessment of pain?   [ ] Yes   [ ] No

5. If desired outcomes were not achieved, is there evidence of action taken?   [ ] Yes   [ ] No

6. Is there evidence that preventative interventions related to possible side effects were implemented?   [ ] Yes   [ ] No

7. If side-effects related to pain interventions occurred, is there evidence of prompt treatment?   [ ] Yes   [ ] No
           [ ] Not applicable

8. If referral to the multidisciplinary team or community care was necessary:
    (a) Was it made at an appropriate stage in the care of the patient?   [ ] Yes   [ ] No
           [ ] Not applicable

    (b) Is there evidence that appropriate information was clearly communicated to the appropriate people?   [ ] Yes   [ ] No
           [ ] Not applicable

NURSING

9. Is there evidence that the patient's pain(s) was (were) minimized   [ ] Yes   [ ] No
   while in hospital?

10. Is there evidence that the patient's pain(s) was (were) relieved   [ ] Yes   [ ] No
    while in hospital?

Nursing Standards of Care

STOMA CARE
PATIENT OPINION

The nursing staff at The Royal Marsden Hospital are constantly trying to improve the service they provide for patients. It is of enormous help to have the views of patients to help us do this and we would like to collect some information from you about your experience of the care the nurses have provided.

We would be very grateful if you would be willing to complete this questionnaire and return it in the envelope provided. The information you provide is confidential and will be treated accordingly.

Thank you for taking the time to complete this questionnaire

1. Did you feel that you received adequate information, prior to being admitted to the ward, about what to expect while in hospital?   [ ] Yes [ ] No

   If no, what information would have been more helpful?

2. Did you feel that your work, leisure and social activities were considered before the site for the stoma was chosen?

   Work   [ ] Yes [ ] No
   Leisure activities   [ ] Yes [ ] No
   Social activities   [ ] Yes [ ] No

   Please comment if you would like to:

3. Did you feel that you were given an accurate picture of what it would be like to have a stoma?   [ ] Yes [ ] No

   If no, how could you have been better prepared?

4. Did you receive a booklet on stomas?   [ ] Yes [ ] No

   If yes, did you find it helpful?   [ ] Yes [ ] No

   If no, what would have made it more useful?

NURSING

5. Did you feel that you had enough privacy when caring for your stoma?　　[ ] Yes　[ ] No

If no, how could we have improved this for you?

6. If you wanted your family to be involved in caring for your stoma, were they given the opportunity and support to do so?

Opportunity　　　　　　　　　　　　　　　　　　　　[ ] Yes　[ ] No
Support　　　　　　　　　　　　　　　　　　　　　　[ ] Yes　[ ] No

Please comment if you would like to:

7. After your operation, did you feel that you had a choice about which stoma product was the most suitable for you?　　[ ] Yes　[ ] No

Please comment if you would like to:

8. Did you feel that you received enough support and teaching to care for your stoma at home?

Support　　　　　　　　　　　　　　　　　　　　　　[ ] Yes　[ ] No
Teaching　　　　　　　　　　　　　　　　　　　　　　[ ] Yes　[ ] No

If no, what more would have been helpful?

9. Were you given enough details about how to obtain equipment when you were at home?　　[ ] Yes　[ ] No

If no, what further information would have been useful?

10. If problems with your stoma occur at home, do you know what to do?　　[ ] Yes　[ ] No

Please comment if you would like to:

11. Overall, did you feel satisfied with the nursing care that you received?　　[ ] Yes　[ ] No

Please comment if you would like to:

12. What did you find most helpful about the care provided for your stoma?

13. What did you find the least helpful about the care provided for your stoma?

Are there any other comments that you would like to make?

Thank you again for completing this questionnaire

STOMA CARE
NURSE OPINION

STANDARD STATEMENT

Patients who have a stoma, either permanent or temporary, will be offered support, information and practical help to enable both themselves (and their families) to care safely and independently for their stoma whilst in the hospital setting and on their return home. Nursing care will be directed towards providing a comprehensive rehabilitation programme to enable patients to integrate wherever possible the management of the stoma into their everyday lives.

1. Do you consider that you had access to all the members of the multidisciplinary team that you required to achieve this standard?   [ ] Yes [ ] No

   If not, who was not available and what impact did it have on the care that you were aiming to provide?

2. Do you consider that you had access to the equipment necessary to achieve this standard?   [ ] Yes [ ] No

   If no, what was not available and why?

3. Do you consider that you had access to the environment necessary to achieve this standard?   [ ] Yes [ ] No

   If no, what was unavailable or unsuitable and why?

4. Do you consider that you had access to educational and managerial support to achieve this standard?
   Educational support   [ ] Yes [ ] No
   Managerial support   [ ] Yes [ ] No

   If no, what aspect(s) were lacking and how did this impact on the care that you were aiming to provide?

5. Do you feel that you were able to follow the professional practice described in the standard?   [ ] Yes [ ] No

   If no, which sections were you unable to follow and why?

6. Did you receive adequate information (via report, the careplan and documentation) to maintain continuity of care when you were taking care of the patient?   [ ] Yes [ ] No

   If no, what information were you lacking?

7. Did you consider that at discharge the patient was able to care competently for their stoma?   [ ] Yes [ ] No

NURSING

If no, why do you consider that the patient was unable to care competently for their stoma?

8. Do you consider that the patient was satisfied with his/her care? [ ] Yes [ ] No

If no, why do you feel that the patient was not satisfied?

9. Overall, do you feel satisfied with the care that you delivered to the patient? [ ] Yes [ ] No

If no, why were you not satisfied?

Do you have any other comments you would like to make?

STOMA CARE DOCUMENTATION

STANDARD STATEMENT

Patients who have a stoma, either permanent or temporary, will be offered support, information and practical help to enable both themselves and their families to care safely and independently for their stoma whilst in the hospital setting and on their return home. Nursing care will be directed towards providing a comprehensive rehabilitation programme to enable patients to integrate wherever possible the management of the stoma into their everyday lives.

1. Is there evidence that the following were assessed?

	Pre-operatively	Post-operatively
(a) The patient's knowledge of what a stoma is?	[ ] Yes [ ] No	[ ] Yes [ ] No
(b) The patient's feelings related to the stoma?	[ ] Yes [ ] No	[ ] Yes [ ] No
(c) The patient's wishes for his/her family to be involved in care?	[ ] Yes [ ] No	[ ] Yes [ ] No
(d) The patient's work activities?	[ ] Yes [ ] No	[ ] Yes [ ] No
– leisure activities?	[ ] Yes [ ] No	[ ] Yes [ ] No
– social activities?	[ ] Yes [ ] No	[ ] Yes [ ] No
(e) Physical limitations which may affect the patients ability to care for their stoma?	[ ] Yes [ ] No	[ ] Yes [ ] No
(f) The patient's needs for information?	[ ] Yes [ ] No	[ ] Yes [ ] No
(g) The family's needs for information?	[ ] Yes [ ] No	[ ] Yes [ ] No
(h) Condition of the stoma?		[ ] Yes [ ] No

2. Were the areas of need identified in the assessment addressed in the care plan?   [ ] Yes [ ] No

3. Is there evidence that the patient was given an information booklet?   [ ] Yes [ ] No

4. Who sited the intended position of the stoma?

5. Was the type and size of the stoma care equipment noted?   [ ] Yes [ ] No

6. Is there evidence that care was evaluated?   [ ] Yes [ ] No

7. If needs for change in care were identified, is there evidence that they were acted upon?   [ ] Yes [ ] No

8. Was the patient referred to a stoma care nurse prior to discharge?   [ ] Yes [ ] No

9. Was the patient offered advice about the available voluntary services and support groups?   [ ] Yes [ ] No

10. On discharge, is there evidence that the patient received enough support and information to be able to care competently for their stoma at home and facilitate the management of the stoma into their everyday life?   [ ] Yes [ ] No

Occupational Therapy
Standards of Care

GENERAL STANDARD
PATIENT OPINION

The occupational therapy staff at The Royal Marsden Hospital are constantly trying to improve the service they provide for patients. It is of enormous help to have the views of patients to help us do this and we would like to collect some information from you about your experience of the care the occupational therapists have provided.

We would be very grateful if you would be willing to complete this questionnaire and return it in the envelope provided. The information you provide is confidential and will be treated accordingly.

Thank you for taking the time to complete this questionnaire

1. Were you clear about why the occupational therapist was asked   [ ] Yes   [ ] No
    to see you?

    Please comment if you would like to:

2. Did you have an opportunity to discuss your practical needs, e.g.   [ ] Yes   [ ] No
    how you would manage at home, with the occupational therapist?

    Please comment if you would like to:

3. Did the advice, information and/or practical help that you
    received from the occupational therapist enable you to be more
    independent?
    Advice   [ ] Yes   [ ] No
                                                                        [ ] Not
                                                                            applicable

    Information   [ ] Yes   [ ] No
                                                                        [ ] Not
                                                                            applicable

    Practical help   [ ] Yes   [ ] No
                                                                        [ ] Not
                                                                            applicable

If no, what would have further helped you?

4. If you received any equipment from the occupational therapist,
(a) Did you find it useful?

[ ] Yes [ ] No
[ ] Not
applicable

(b) Did you receive enough information to put it to use easily?

[ ] Yes [ ] No
[ ] Not
applicable

(c) Did you receive it promptly?

[ ] Yes [ ] No
[ ] Not
applicable

If no, please comment as to any difficulties you had:

5. If you received any written information from the occupational therapist, did you find it understandable and helpful?
[ ] Did not receive any written information
Understandable
Helpful

[ ] Yes [ ] No
[ ] Yes [ ] No

If no, what would have made it more useful?

6. If you attended relaxation classes run by occupational therapy did you find them useful?

[ ] Yes [ ] No
[ ] Not
applicable

If no, what would have made them more useful?

7. If you had a 'home visit' from the occupational therapist:
(a) Did you understand the reasons for it?

[ ] Yes [ ] No
[ ] Not
applicable

(b) Was it helpful?

[ ] Yes [ ] No
[ ] Not
applicable

Please comment if you would like to:

8. If complications were to arise related to managing independently at home, do you know who to contact?

[ ] Yes [ ] No

Please comment if you would like to:

9. Overall, did you feel that the occupational therapist helped to prepare you for returning home?

[ ] Yes [ ] No

Please comment if you would like to:

10. Overall, were you satisfied with the advice/treatment offered by   [ ] Yes [ ] No
the occupational therapist?

Please comment if you would like to:

11. What did you find the most helpful about the treatment offered by
the occupational therapist?

12. What did you find the least helpful about the treatment offered by
the occupational therapist?

Are there any other comments you would like to make?

Thank you for taking the time to complete this questionnaire

OCCUPATIONAL THERAPY

GENERAL STANDARD
OCCUPATIONAL THERAPIST OPINION

STANDARD STATEMENT

Occupational therapy is directed towards enabling patients to achieve and maintain their optimum level of independence in all areas of their daily lives.

1. Did you consider that the timing of the referral to Occupational Therapy was appropriate?　　　　　　　　　　　　[ ] Yes　[ ] No

If no, why was it not an appropriate time?

2. Do you consider that you had access to all the members of the multidisciplinary team that you required to achieve this standard?　　　　　　　　　　　　　　　　[ ] Yes　[ ] No

If not, who was not available, and how did this impact on the care you were aiming to provide?

3. Do you consider that you had access to the equipment necessary to achieve this standard?　　　　　　　　　　　　[ ] Yes　[ ] No

If no, what was not available and why?

4. Do you consider that you had access to the environment necessary to achieve this standard?　　　　　　　　　　　[ ] Yes　[ ] No

If no, what was unavailable or unsuitable and why?

5. Do you consider that you had access to the educational and managerial support necessary to achieve this standard?

Educational support　　　　　　　　　　　　　　　[ ] Yes　[ ] No

Managerial support　　　　　　　　　　　　　　　[ ] Yes　[ ] No

If no, what aspect(s) were not met and how did this impact on the care you were aiming to provide?

6. Do you feel that you were able to follow the professional practice described in the standard?　　　　　　　　　　　[ ] Yes　[ ] No

If no, which sections were you unable to follow and why?

7. Do you consider that you received adequate information (via report, care plans and documentation) to maintain continuity of care while caring for this patient?　　　　　　　　　[ ] Yes　[ ] No

If no, what information were you lacking?

8. Do you consider that the patient achieved their optimum level of   [ ] Yes [ ] No
   independence?

   If no, why do you feel they were unable to achieve this?

9. Do you consider that the patient and family were able to manage
   safely and independently in the community?
   Safely   [ ] Yes [ ] No
   Independently   [ ] Yes [ ] No

   If no, please comment

10. Do you consider that the patient was satisfied with their care?   [ ] Yes [ ] No

    If no, why do you feel that the patient was not satisfied?

11. Overall, do you feel satisfied with the care that you delivered to   [ ] Yes [ ] No
    the patient?

    If no, why were you not satisfied?

    Do you have any other comments you would like to make?

OCCUPATIONAL THERAPY

GENERAL STANDARD DOCUMENTATION

| STANDARD STATEMENT |

Occupational therapy is directed towards enabling patients to achieve and maintain their optimum level of independence in all areas of their daily lives.

1. Is there evidence that the patient was contacted within 72 hours of referral? [ ] Yes [ ] No

2. Is there evidence that the following was assessed?
(a) The patient's medical history [ ] Yes [ ] No
(b) The patient's view of current situation [ ] Yes [ ] No
(c) Functional ability related to ADL's [ ] Yes [ ] No
(d) Functional ability related to mobility [ ] Yes [ ] No
(e) Potential need for pressure area care [ ] Yes [ ] No
(f) Psychological state [ ] Yes [ ] No
(g) The patient's social situation [ ] Yes [ ] No

3. Were problem areas clearly listed in the documentation? [ ] Yes [ ] No

4. Were the treatment aims reflective of the problems identified? [ ] Yes [ ] No

5. Is there evidence that care was evaluated? [ ] Yes [ ] No

6. If outcomes were not achieved, is there evidence of action taken? [ ] Yes [ ] No
[ ] Not applicable

7. Is there evidence that at discharge the patient had reached their maximum potential? [ ] Yes [ ] No

8. Is there evidence that at discharge the patient and family would be able to manage independently in the community? [ ] Yes [ ] No

9. If a formal assessment (e.g. for Social Services, Disability Services Centre, Disablement Resettlement Officer etc.) was necessary, was a written report sent to the appropriate person? [ ] Yes [ ] No
[ ] Not applicable

10. If referral to members of the multidisciplinary team or community care was necessary,

(a) Was it made at an appropriate stage? [ ] Yes [ ] No
                                          [ ] Not
                                              applicable

(b) Is there evidence that the appropriate information was clearly   [ ] Yes [ ] No
    communicated?   [ ] Not
                                                                         applicable

OCCUPATIONAL THERAPY

Physiotherapy Standards of Care

BREAST SURGERY PATIENT OPINION

The physiotherapy staff at The Royal Marsden Hospital are constantly trying to improve the service they provide for patients. It is of enormous help to have the views of patients to help us do this and we would like to collect some information from you about your experience of the care the physiotherapists have provided.

We would be very grateful if you would be willing to complete this questionnaire and return it in the envelope provided. The information you provide is confidential and will be treated accordingly.

Thank you for taking the time to complete this questionnaire

1. Did you understand why the physiotherapist was asked to see you?

   Please comment if you would like to: [ ] Yes [ ] No

2. Were you given enough information and support to perform the physiotherapy exercises on your own?
   Information   [ ] Yes [ ] No
   Support   [ ] Yes [ ] No

   If no, what could the physiotherapist have done that would have been more helpful?

3. Did you find the advice or exercise sheets helpful?   [ ] Yes [ ] No
                                                                          [ ] Did not
   Please comment on any difficulties you experienced: receive any

4. If you had the lymph nodes removed from your armpit (axilla),   [ ] Yes [ ] No
   were you given a leaflet and advice about what you need to do in   [ ] Not
   order to prevent any swelling in your arm?   applicable

   Please comment on whether you found the leaflet and advice helpful:

5. Did you receive adequate advice and support from the physiotherapist about returning to your home, work and leisure activities?

Advice [ ] Yes [ ] No

Support [ ] Yes [ ] No

If no, what further information would have been more helpful?

6. Did you feel that you had confidence in the physiotherapist? [ ] Yes [ ] No

Please comment if you would like to:

7. Overall, do you feel satisfied with the care and information that the physiotherapist provided to help you regain the use of your arm?

Care [ ] Yes [ ] No

Information [ ] Yes [ ] No

If no, what could be improved to provide a better service for you?

8. What did you find most helpful about the physiotherapy service provided?

9. What did you find the least helpful about the physiotherapy service provided?

Are there any other comments you would like to make?

Thank you once again for completing this questionnaire

BREAST SURGERY
PHYSIOTHERAPIST OPINION

STANDARD STATEMENT

Physiotherapy for patients who have undergone *either* surgical dissection of the axillary nodes with or without wide local excision of the breast lump, *or* mastectomy with or without breast reconstruction is directed towards enabling patients, on discharge from physiotherapy, to continue their exercises and understand the instruction that will enable them, firstly, to regain maximum function ability of the upper limb ipsilateral to the breast surgery and, secondly, to minimize the risk of developing post-operative lymphoedema.

1. Do you consider that you had access to all the members of the multidisciplinary team that you required to achieve this standard?   [ ] Yes [ ] No

If not, how did this impact on the care that you were aiming to provide?

2. If you received the referral from another member of the multidisciplinary team, do you consider that:
(a) It was made at an appropriate time   [ ] Yes [ ] No
(b) You received adequate information   [ ] Yes [ ] No
(c) Recommendations which had implications for other health care professionals were followed through   [ ] Yes [ ] No
[ ] Not applicable

3. Do you consider that you had access to the equipment necessary to achieve this standard?   [ ] Yes [ ] No

If no, what was not available and why?

4. Do you consider that you had access to the environment necessary to achieve this standard?   [ ] Yes [ ] No

If no, what was unavailable or unsuitable and why?

5. Do you consider that you had access to educational and managerial support to achieve this standard?
Educational support   [ ] Yes [ ] No
Managerial support   [ ] Yes [ ] No

If no, which aspect(s) were lacking – and how did this impact on the care you were aiming to provide?

6. Do you feel that you were able to follow the professional practice described in the standard?   [ ] Yes [ ] No

If no, which sections were you unable to follow and why?

7. Do you consider that the patient understood the information and advice that you provided about exercises and the prevention of lymphoedema? [ ] Yes [ ] No

If no, why did you feel that the patient did not understand?

8. Do you consider that the patient will be able to regain maximal functioning of the affected arm/shoulder? [ ] Yes [ ] No

If no, why do you feel that she is unable to achieve this?

9. Do you consider that the patient was satisfied with her physiotherapy treatment? [ ] Yes [ ] No

If no, why did you feel that the patient was not satisfied?

10. Overall, do you feel satisfied with the care that you delivered to the patient? [ ] Yes [ ] No

If no, why were you not satisfied?

Are there any other comments that you would like to make?

BREAST SURGERY DOCUMENTATION

STANDARD STATEMENT

Physiotherapy for patients who have undergone *either* surgical dissection of the axillary nodes with or without wide local excision of the breast lump, *or* mastectomy with or without breast reconstruction is directed towards enabling patients, on discharge from physiotherapy, to continue their exercises and understand the instruction that will enable them, firstly, to regain maximum function ability of the upper limb ipsilateral to the breast surgery and, secondly, to minimize the risk of developing post-operative lymphoedema.

1. Pre-operatively, was the patient assessed by a physiotherapist for all items listed in the standard of care?　　[ ] Yes　[ ] No

If no, which were omitted?

2. Was the patient assessed post-operatively for all the items listed in the standard of care?　　[ ] Yes　[ ] No

If no, which were omitted?

3. Did the treatment plan address areas of need identified in the pre/post operative assessment?　　[ ] Yes　[ ] No

4. Was there evidence of evaluation of care provided?　　[ ] Yes　[ ] No

5. If needs for change in care were identified, is there evidence that action was taken?　　[ ] Yes　[ ] No

6. If on discharge from physiotherapy, the patient's functional ability was not at pre-operative level, was further advice given and/or treatment arranged to enable the patient to achieve this?

Advice　　[ ] Yes　[ ] No

Treatment　　[ ] Yes　[ ] No

7. On discharge from physiotherapy, had the patient been given advice to ensure that he/she knew how to prevent the development of lymphoedema in the future?　　[ ] Yes　[ ] No

8. If referral to the multidisciplinary team or another physiotherapy department was deemed necessary:

(a) Was it made at an appropriate stage in the care of the patient?　　[ ] Yes　[ ] No　[ ] Not applicable

(b) Is there evidence that appropriate information was clearly communicated to the appropriate people?　　[ ] Yes　[ ] No　[ ] Not applicable

Speech and Language Therapy
Standards of Care

LARYNGECTOMY
PATIENT OPINION

The speech and language therapists at The Royal Marsden Hospital are constantly trying to improve the service they provide for patients. It is of enormous help to have the views of patients to help us do this and we would like to collect some information from you about your experience of the care the speech and language therapists have provided.

We would be very grateful if you would be willing to complete this questionnaire and return it in the envelope provided. The information you provide is confidential and will be treated accordingly.

Thank you for taking the time to complete this questionnaire

1. Did you understand why the speech and language therapist was asked to see you?   [ ] Yes   [ ] No

   Please comment if you would like to:

2. Do you consider you were given an accurate picture of how you would communicate after your operation?   [ ] Yes   [ ] No

   If no, what would have given you a clearer picture?

3. Did you find the Patient Information Booklet 'Laryngectomy' helpful?   [ ] Yes   [ ] No
   [ ] Did not
   receive a
   booklet

   What would have made it more useful?

   If you had a voice valve fitted please answer question 4: if not, please move on to question 5.

4. (a) On the day you had your valve fitted, did you have to wait prior to seeing the speech and language therapist?   [ ] Yes   [ ]No

   If yes, how long did you have to wait?

   (b) Did you receive enough information and practical help to use your valve?

Information   [ ] Yes   [ ] No
Practical help   [ ] Yes   [ ] No
(c) Do you feel confident in using your valve voice?   [ ] Yes   [ ] No

If no to either 'b' or 'c', how could we have helped you further?

If you did not have a voice valve fitted, please answer question 5.
Otherwise, please move on to question 6.

5. (a) Do you feel that the options available for communicating following your operation were clearly explained to you?   [ ] Yes   [ ] No

(b) Did you receive enough information and practical help to use the communication method you have chosen?

Information   [ ] Yes   [ ] No
Practical help   [ ] Yes   [ ] No

(c) Do you feel confident in using the communication method you have chosen?   [ ] Yes   [ ] No

If no to any of the above, what would have helped you further?

6. If your family wanted to be involved in care, were they given enough information, support and practical advice to do so?   [ ] Yes   [ ] No
     [ ] Did not wish to be involved

Please comment if you would like to:

7. If questions arose while you were at home, did you know who to contact?   [ ] Yes   [ ] No

If no, what further information would have been more helpful?

8. Did you feel that you had confidence in the speech and language therapist?   [ ] Yes   [ ] No

Please comment if you would like to:

9. Overall, do you feel satisfied with the care, advice and information that the speech and language therapist provided?   [ ] Yes   [ ] No

If no, what could be improved to provide a better service for you?

10. What did you find most helpful about the care provided?

11. What did you find the least helpful about the care provided?

Are there any other comments you would like to make?

Thank you once again for completing this questionnaire

LARYNGECTOMY
SPEECH AND LANGUAGE THERAPIST OPINION

STANDARD STATEMENT

Speech and language therapy for the patient undergoing laryngectomy aims to ensure the patient has a clear understanding of the anatomical and physiological changes involved, that the patient is aware of the long term options for communication and that help is offered for any swallowing difficulties which might arise.

1. Do you consider that you had access to all the members of the multidisciplinary team that you required to achieve this standard? [ ] Yes [ ] No

   If no, how did this impact on the care that you were aiming to provide?

2. If you received the referral from another member of the multi-disciplinary team, do you consider that
   (a) it was made at an appropriate time [ ] Yes [ ] No
   (b) you received adequate and clear information [ ] Yes [ ] No
   (c) recommendations which had implications for other health care professionals were followed through [ ] Yes [ ] No [ ] Not applicable

3. Do you consider that you had access to the equipment necessary to achieve this standard? [ ] Yes [ ] No

   If no, what was not available and why?

4. Do you consider that you had access to the environment necessary to achieve this standard? [ ] Yes [ ] No

   If no, what was unavailable or unsuitable and why?

5. Do you consider that you had access to educational and managerial support to achieve this standard?
   Educational support [ ] Yes [ ] No
   Managerial support [ ] Yes [ ] No

   If no, which aspect(s) were lacking – and how did this impact on the care you were aiming to provide?

6. Do you feel that you were able to follow the professional practice described in the standard? [ ] Yes [ ] No

   If no, which sections were you unable to follow and why?

7. Do you consider that everything possible was offered to enable the patient to communicate at an optimal level? [ ] Yes [ ] No

If no, why did you feel this was not accomplished?

8. Do you consider that the patient achieved their optimal level of communication?　　[ ] Yes　[ ] No

If no, why do you feel that he/she did not achieve this?

9. Do you consider that the patient was satisfied with his/her speech and language therapy treatment?　　[ ] Yes　[ ] No

If no, why did you feel that the patient was not satisfied?

10. Overall, do you feel satisfied with the care that you delivered to the patient?　　[ ] Yes　[ ] No

If no, why were you not satisfied?

Are there any other comments that you would like to make?

LARYNGECTOMY DOCUMENTATION

STANDARD STATEMENT

Speech and language therapy for the patient undergoing laryngectomy aims to ensure the patient has a clear understanding of the anatomical and physiological changes involved, that the patient is aware of the long-term options for communication and that help is offered for any swallowing difficulties which might arise.

1. Pre-operatively, is there evidence that the following were assessed?
   (a) The patient's communication skills   [ ] Yes   [ ] No
   (b) The patient's adjustment to the diagnosis   [ ] Yes   [ ] No
   (c) The patient's body awareness   [ ] Yes   [ ] No
   (d) The patient's vision   [ ] Yes   [ ] No
   (e) The patient's hearing   [ ] Yes   [ ] No
   (f) The patient's dexterity   [ ] Yes   [ ] No
   (g) The implications of the medical plan   [ ] Yes   [ ] No

2. If a valve was to be fitted were the valve details and post-operative complications recorded?   [ ] Yes   [ ] No

   If no, what was omitted?

3. If a valve was not fitted is there evidence that other options for communication were explored?   [ ] Yes   [ ] No

4. Did the treatment plan address areas of need identified in the assessment?   [ ] Yes   [ ] No

5. Was there evidence of evaluation of care provided?   [ ] Yes   [ ] No

6. If needs for change in care were identified, is there evidence that action was taken?   [ ] Yes   [ ] No

7. Is there evidence that the patient had achieved the optimum communication level for him/her?   [ ] Yes   [ ] No

8. If referral to the multidisciplinary team or another speech and language therapy department was necessary:
   (a) Was it made at an appropriate stage in the care of the patient?   [ ] Yes   [ ] No   [ ] Not applicable

   (b) Is there evidence that appropriate information was clearly communicated to the appropriate people?   [ ] Yes   [ ] No   [ ] Not applicable

Index